The Anti-Inflammatory Cookbook For Beginners 2024

Discover the Easy Path to Wellness With Delicious Recipes to Soothe Your Body and Spark Your Vitality.

Table Of Content

Introduction

Overview Of Inflammation And The Influence Of Anti-Inflammatory Foods

The body's normal biological reaction to adverse stimuli like viruses, injuries, or poisons is inflammation. It is an essential component of the immune system's defensive mechanism and starts a chain reaction of cellular and biochemical events to get rid of the danger and encourage recovery. However, persistent or unchecked inflammation may be a factor in a number of medical conditions and have a detrimental effect on general health, especially in elderly people.

The development and progression of several age-related disorders, including cardiovascular disease, arthritis, diabetes, Alzheimer's disease, and certain kinds of cancer, are now understood to be significantly influenced by chronic inflammation. Additionally, it might worsen pre-existing medical disorders and cause seniors' physical and cognitive abilities to deteriorate. Therefore, it is critical to develop strategies for controlling and reducing chronic inflammation if you want to encourage senior citizens to live healthy, extended lives.

Adopting an anti-inflammatory diet, which emphasizes the intake of foods that have anti-inflammatory characteristics and help modify the body's inflammatory response, is a potent weapon in the battle against chronic inflammation. Foods that are anti-inflammatory have the capability to regulate the immune system by promoting the synthesis of anti-inflammatory substances while reducing the development of pro-inflammatory molecules.

Generally speaking, anti-inflammatory foods are high in minerals, antioxidants, and phytochemicals, all of which combine to fight oxidative stress and reduce inflammation. Omega-3 fatty acids, polyphenols, carotenoids, vitamins, minerals, fiber, and polyphenols are a few important ingredients in these meals. By including these foods in their diets, seniors may be able to reduce their chance of developing chronic illnesses, strengthen their immune systems, and improve their general wellbeing.

An anti-inflammatory diet for elderly has advantages beyond just reducing inflammation. Numerous meals that are suggested are also linked to better cardiovascular health, better digestive function, and healthier weight control, as well as a decreased risk of age-related cognitive decline. An anti-inflammatory diet supports the consumption of whole, minimally processed foods while avoiding the intake of refined carbohydrates, harmful fats, and artificial additives. As a result, following an anti-inflammatory diet often results in an overall increase in nutritional quality.

While an anti-inflammatory diet may be advantageous for seniors, it is crucial to remember that there is no one-size-fits-all solution. Individual health problems and dietary choices, as well as nutritional demands, should be taken into account. It is advised to get advice from a medical expert or qualified dietician to guarantee individualized advice and to address any particular problems.

We want to provide elders with a range of wholesome dishes in this cookbook that are created to include a variety of anti-inflammatory foods and components. Our recipes are created with care to be delicious, simple to make, and fit for seniors' specific nutritional needs. Each dish focuses on using anti-inflammatory foods to enhance general health and wellbeing, from invigorating breakfast alternatives to filling main meals, healthy snacks, and decadent desserts.

Seniors may actively participate in controlling inflammation, lowering their chance of developing chronic illnesses, and fostering a vibrant and meaningful life by embracing the potential of anti-inflammatory foods and including them in regular meals. Let this cookbook serve as your guide to discovering the world of delectable and healthy meals that will excite your palate and aid in your quest for improved health.

Remember that the decisions we make in the kitchen are the first step in achieving maximum wellness. Let's begin this culinary journey together and learn how anti-inflammatory meals for seniors may improve lives.

Chapter 1:

An Overview of the Anti-Inflammatory Diet

An anti-inflammatory diet has gained popularity in recent years due to its potential health advantages, especially in the management of chronic inflammation. Chronic inflammation has been linked to a variety of health problems, including heart disease, arthritis, diabetes, and even certain kinds of cancer. The anti-inflammatory diet tries to decrease inflammation in the body by encouraging the use of anti-inflammatory foods and limiting the consumption of items that might cause inflammation.

The anti-inflammatory diet's ideas are based on the concept that particular foods may either stimulate or reduce inflammation in the body. We may impact our body's inflammatory response and perhaps lessen the chance of acquiring chronic illnesses connected with inflammation by making thoughtful food choices.

So, how exactly does an anti-inflammatory diet work? Let's look at the basic ideas and advantages of this nutritional strategy.

Anti-Inflammatory Diet Principles:

Emphasize whole, plant-based foods: The anti-inflammatory diet is built on whole, minimally processed plant foods. Fruits, vegetables, whole grains, legumes, nuts, and seeds are examples. These foods are high in antioxidants, vitamins, minerals, and fiber, all of which help to reduce inflammation.

The anti-inflammatory diet promotes the use of good fats such as those found in olive oil, avocados, nuts, and seeds. These lipids have a high concentration of omega-3 fatty acids, which have been demonstrated to alleviate inflammation in the body.

Include Fatty Fish: Fatty fish such as salmon, mackerel, sardines, and trout are high in omega-3 fatty acids. Omega-3 fatty acids have powerful anti-inflammatory properties and may help balance the omega-6 to omega-3 ratio in the body, which is critical for inflammation regulation.

Processed foods, such as those heavy in added sugars, refined carbohydrates, and unhealthy fats, are known to increase inflammation. These processed and highly processed foods, according to the anti-inflammatory diet, should be limited or avoided since they may lead to chronic inflammation and other health problems.

Choose Lean Protein: The plan recommends eating lean protein sources such as chicken, fish, lentils, and tofu. These protein sources have a lower saturated fat content than red meat and may deliver vital amino acids without adding excessive inflammation-promoting components.

Anti-Inflammatory Herbs and Spices: Many herbs and spices have anti-inflammatory qualities. Spices such as turmeric, ginger, garlic, cinnamon, and chili peppers may be added to meals to provide taste while also having possible anti-inflammatory effects.

Anti-Inflammatory Diet Advantages:

Reduced Chronic Inflammation: Adopting an anti-inflammatory diet may result in a decrease in chronic inflammation indicators in the body. As a result, the risk of acquiring chronic illnesses connected with inflammation may be reduced.

Heart Health Improvement: Chronic inflammation is a proven risk factor for heart disease. By lowering inflammation, improving blood lipid profiles, and maintaining appropriate blood pressure levels, an anti-inflammatory diet may enhance heart health.

Management of Joint Health and Arthritis: Inflammation is a major factor in joint pain and arthritis. With its focus on nutrient-rich foods and omega-3 fatty acids, the anti-inflammatory diet may help ease joint discomfort, reduce swelling, and enhance overall joint health.

Improved Gut Health: The gut and its microbiome have a large influence on overall health, including inflammatory levels. A fiber-rich diet rich in fruits, vegetables, and whole grains helps maintain healthy gut flora, lowering inflammation and improving digestive health.

Obesity and excess body weight have been linked to increased inflammation in the body. Individuals who follow an anti-inflammatory diet might make better dietary choices, perhaps leading to weight loss or weight control and a decrease in inflammation.

While the anti-inflammatory diet shows promise in terms of increasing health and reducing inflammation, it is not a panace It should be seen as a component of a comprehensive approach to general well-being that includes regular exercise, stress management, and appropriate sleep.

To summarize, the anti-inflammatory diet is a dietary strategy that emphasizes the consumption of complete, nutrient-dense foods while avoiding pro-inflammatory items. Individuals who adhere to the principles of this diet may have decreased chronic inflammation, improved heart health, joint health, gut health, and better weight control. A healthcare practitioner or qualified dietitian may give tailored direction and help in implementing an anti-inflammatory diet to realize its potential advantages.

How a Diet Low in Inflammation Promotes Senior Health

Our bodies change as we age, and the chance of developing chronic illnesses and age-related disorders rises. An important part of our body's defensive systems is inflammation, a normal immunological reaction to damage or illness. On the other hand, persistent inflammation may be harmful to general health, especially for elderly people. Fortunately, consuming a diet low in inflammation may greatly increase general wellbeing and support elderly health.

Reducing the Risk of Chronic Illnesses: Many age-related illnesses, including cardiovascular disease, diabetes, arthritis, neurological disorders, and certain kinds of cancer, are intimately linked to chronic inflammation. Senior citizens may lower their chance of developing these diseases by switching to a diet low in inflammation. Consuming nutrient-rich, whole foods is emphasized in the anti-inflammatory diet, while avoiding processed foods, refined carbohydrates, and bad fats is discouraged. By reducing inflammatory signals in the body, this strategy promotes a more healthy aging process.

Supporting Joint Health: For older people, arthritis and joint discomfort are prevalent worries. Joint inflammation may cause soreness, edema, and stiffness. Seniors who eat a diet low in inflammatory foods, such as fatty fish high in omega-3 fatty acids, colorful fruits and vegetables high in antioxidants, and spices like turmeric and ginger with anti-inflammatory qualities, might have less joint inflammation. These food options may ease joint discomfort, increase mobility, and promote general joint health.

Maintaining a Healthy Weight: Obesity and excess weight may cause chronic inflammation and raise your chance of developing a number of illnesses, including diabetes, heart disease, and several types of cancer. By putting an emphasis on whole foods, lean proteins, fiber-rich fruits and vegetables, and healthy fats, a diet low in inflammation supports weight control. These food selections may help seniors' metabolic health, reduce inflammation, and achieve weight reduction or weight maintenance.

Enhancing Cognitive Function: Alzheimer's and Parkinson's disease are two important causes of worry for elderly people, as are age-related cognitive decline and neurodegenerative disorders. Cognitive impairment may be exacerbated by persistent brain inflammation. However, evidence indicates that consuming an anti-inflammatory diet high in antioxidants, omega-3 fatty acids, vitamins, and minerals may help safeguard brain health, slow the deterioration of cognition, and maintain cognitive performance in older people.

Improving Digestive Health: Aging may cause changes in the digestive system, including decreased synthesis of digestive enzymes, sluggish gut motility, and a higher risk of gastrointestinal problems. In irritable bowel syndrome (IBS) and inflammatory bowel disease

(IBD), gut inflammation may be a factor in digestive diseases. Seniors should include items that promote gut health in their anti-inflammatory diets, such as probiotics found in fermented foods like yogurt and kefir, fiber-rich whole grains, and gastrointestinal-soothing herbs and spices. These food options may help to maintain a balanced gut flora, enhance digestion, and lessen digestive system inflammation.

Immune system bolstering: As we age, our immune systems become less effective, leaving older people more vulnerable to infections and diseases. Immune system performance might be further hampered by chronic inflammation. Seniors may provide their bodies with the vital nutrients they need to build a strong immune system by eating a diet low in inflammation. Fruits, vegetables, whole grains, lean meats, and healthy fats are nutrient-dense foods that are rich with vitamins, minerals, and antioxidants that support immune function and decrease inflammation.

Increasing Vitality and Energy: Seniors often feel low energy and weariness. These symptoms may be exacerbated by inflammation. A diet that reduces inflammation places a priority on nutrient-dense foods that provide you with long-lasting energy, such as complex carbs, lean proteins, and healthy fats. Seniors who feed their bodies with these nutrient-dense foods may notice an improvement in their general quality of life, energy levels, and vitality.

Finally, adopting a diet low in inflammation may significantly improve the health of seniors. Seniors may lower their chance of developing chronic illnesses, promote joint health, maintain a healthy weight, improve digestive health, strengthen their immune systems, and experience an increase in energy and vitality by including anti-inflammatory items in their diets. Before making any dietary adjustments, seniors should speak with a healthcare provider or certified dietitian to ensure that their unique requirements and medical circumstances are taken into account. Seniors may improve their well-being and live a healthier, more active life by eating with awareness and knowledge.

Chapter 2

Essential Nutrients For The Management Of Inflammation

The immune system's natural defense against potentially hazardous stimuli like viruses, injuries, or poisons is inflammation. However, prolonged or severe inflammation may lead to the emergence of a number of diseases, such as autoimmune disorders, cardiovascular disease, and arthritis. Happily, eating a diet high in important nutrients may assist control inflammation and advance optimum health. This article examines various essential nutrients with anti-inflammatory qualities and their function in the control of inflammation.

Eicosapentaenoic acid (EPA) and docosahexaenoic acid (DHA), in particular, are two omega-3 fatty acids recognized for their strong anti-inflammatory properties. These fatty acids are widely distributed in foods including walnuts, flaxseeds, chia seeds, and fatty seafood like salmon, mackerel, and sardines. Inflammation is lessened by omega-3 fatty acids through lowering the body's synthesis of pro-inflammatory chemicals such prostaglandins and cytokines. In diseases including rheumatoid arthritis, cardiovascular disease, and inflammatory bowel disease, they have been linked to lower levels of inflammatory markers and better results.

Antioxidants are substances that shield the body's cells from the oxidative damage brought on by free radicals. A surplus of free radicals produced by chronic inflammation may harm cells and fuel more inflammation. Inflammation is diminished as a result of antioxidants' ability to combat these damaging free radicals. Strong antioxidants include beta-carotene, selenium, flavonoids, vitamins C and E, and others. They are present in a broad variety of foods, including berries, citrus fruits, leafy greens, almonds, green tea, and nuts, seeds, and nuts. People may help their bodies fight inflammation by including a range of antioxidant-rich foods in their diet.

Dietary fiber: It has been shown that dietary fiber, especially soluble fiber, has anti-inflammatory properties. By encouraging the development of healthy gut flora, it controls inflammation and aids in immune system regulation. Short-chain fatty acids like butyrate, which are produced by these bacteria, have anti-inflammatory effects. Fiber may also aid in maintaining a healthy weight as extra body fat has been linked to long-term inflammation. Whole grains, legumes, fruits, vegetables, seeds, and legume products are excellent sources of fiber.

Phytochemicals: Phytochemicals are organic substances that are naturally present in plants and have a range of health advantages, including anti-inflammatory properties. Curcumin (found in turmeric), resveratrol (in grapes and red wine), quercetin (in onions and apples), and sulforaphane (in broccoli and cruciferous vegetables) are a few examples of phytochemicals having anti-inflammatory characteristics. The body's inflammatory pathways are inhibited by these substances, which lowers the generation of inflammatory mediators. A vast array of phytochemicals may be obtained from a range of vibrant fruits, vegetables, herbs, and spices, which can also help to reduce inflammation.

Vitamins and minerals: Getting the right amount of vitamins and minerals is essential for keeping the immune system strong and controlling inflammation. Particularly vitamin D has been linked to lowered inflammation and enhanced immunological performance. It controls how different immune cells behave and how anti-inflammatory cytokines are produced. Fatty fish, fortified dairy products, and sun exposure are all natural sources of vitamin D. For the immune system and the control of inflammation, vitamins A, C, E, and zinc are also crucial. They stimulate tissue healing, control immunological responses, and serve as antioxidants. Citrus fruits, leafy greens, nuts, seeds, and lean meats are among the foods that are high in these nutrients.

Probiotics: Probiotics are good bacteria that support a balanced microbiome in the gut. The control of inflammation and the maintenance of a healthy immune system depend heavily on gut flor Probiotics decrease gut permeability, alter immunological responses, and help preserve the integrity of the intestinal barrier. Probiotics may reduce inflammation by promoting a balanced gut microbiot Yogurt, kefir, sauerkraut, kimchi, and other fermented foods are examples of foods high in probiotics.

It's crucial to remember that, although these necessary nutrients have shown promise in controlling inflammation, they work best when included in a balanced diet with a variety of foods. Instead of just using supplements, it is advised to get these nutrients through entire meals. A variety of other beneficial substances that are present in whole meals combine to enhance general health.

Along with include these anti-inflammatory foods in the diet, it's important to have a healthy lifestyle. Regular exercise, enough sleep, stress management, and abstaining from smoking and excessive alcohol intake all help to reduce inflammation and promote overall health.

Individual needs may differ, so it's always advisable to seek advice from a medical professional or registered dietitian before starting any supplementation program or making significant dietary changes, especially for people with particular medical conditions or who are taking medications that may interact with certain nutrients.

In conclusion, vital nutrients are very important in the control of inflammation. Inflammation is reduced and good health is promoted by omega-3 fatty acids, antioxidants, fiber, phytochemicals, vitamins, minerals, and probiotics, among other nutrients. People may help their bodies manage inflammation, thereby lowering their chance of developing chronic illnesses, by adopting a diet high in these nutrients and leading a healthy lifestyle.

Vitamins and minerals: Improving Immune Function and Overall Health

Vitamins and minerals are essential for maintaining and strengthening immune function as well as general health. These important nutrients are required for a variety of biological functions throughout the body, including immune system function. We can assist our bodies' defensive systems and promote good health by maintaining proper vitamin and mineral consumption.

Vitamins are chemical molecules that the body need for growth, development, and general health. Water-soluble vitamins (such as vitamin C and the B vitamins) and fat-soluble vitamins (such as vitamins A, D, E, and K) are divided into two groups. Each vitamin has unique roles and advantages, but particular vitamins stand out when it comes to immune function.

The most well-known immune-boosting vitamin is vitamin It functions as a potent antioxidant, protecting the body from oxidative stress and enhancing immune cell activity. Vitamin C promotes the development of white blood cells, which are necessary for combating infections. It also boosts the activity of natural killer cells, which play an important role in pathogen elimination. Citrus fruits, strawberries, kiwi, bell peppers, and leafy green vegetables are all high in vitamin

B vitamins, such as B6, B9 (folate), and B12, are also essential for immunological function. Vitamin B6 is necessary for the formation of antibodies and white blood cells. It aids the body's capacity to fight infections and helps to regulate inflammation. Poultry, fish, bananas, and chickpeas are all high in vitamin B6. Folate, often known as vitamin B9, is required for the formation and maintenance of cells, particularly immune cells. It may be found in leafy green vegetables, legumes, and fortified grains. Vitamin B12 is required for the synthesis of red blood cells and aids in the maintenance of the immune system's integrity. Meat, fish, and dairy products are great sources of vitamin B12.

Vitamin A is important for immunological health because it promotes the growth and maintenance of the skin and mucous membranes, which serve as barriers against infections. It is also involved in the formation of white blood cells. Animal sources of vitamin A include liver, eggs, and dairy products, as well as plant sources such as carrots, sweet potatoes, and spinach.

Vitamin D, sometimes known as the "sunshine vitamin," is unusual in that it can be produced by our bodies when our skin is exposed to sunlight. Vitamin D is required for the immune system to operate properly. It aids in the regulation of immune cell responses, the generation of antimicrobial peptides, and the absorption of calcium, which is essential for bone health. Fatty fish (such as salmon and mackerel), fortified dairy products, and egg yolks are all good sources of vitamin D.

Vitamin E is an antioxidant that protects the body's cells from free radical damage. It aids in the maintenance of cell membrane integrity and immunological function. Nuts, seeds, vegetable oils, and leafy green vegetables are high in vitamin E.

Minerals, in addition to vitamins, play an important role in immune function and general health. Minerals are inorganic compounds that the body requires in trace quantities for a variety of physiological operations. Zinc, selenium, iron, and copper are all important minerals for immunological function.

Zinc aids in the growth and function of immune cells, as well as the regulation of immunological responses. It is required for the generation of antibodies and promotes the activity of immune-related enzymes. Seafood, pork, legumes, nuts, and seeds are all good sources of zin

Selenium is an antioxidant that is necessary for the immune system to operate properly. It aids in the regulation of inflammation and the activity of immune cells. Brazil nuts, shellfish, whole grains, and eggs are high in selenium.

Iron is required for the formation of red blood cells, which transport oxygen throughout the body. It's also required for immune cell activity. Iron deficiency may decrease immune responses and make you more vulnerable to infections. Iron-rich foods include lean meats, shellfish, beans, lentils, and iron-fortified cereals.

Copper is involved in immune cell growth and function, as well as collagen creation, which is vital for wound healing. Organ meats, seafood, nuts, seeds, and whole grains are all high in copper.

While vitamins and minerals are necessary for immune function, they also operate in tandem with other nutrition and lifestyle variables. A well-balanced and diverse diet rich in fruits, vegetables, whole grains, lean meats, and healthy fats is the best method to guarantee appropriate vitamin and mineral consumption. It is also critical to speak with a healthcare practitioner or qualified dietitian to determine individual nutritional requirements and, if required, supplementation.

Finally, vitamins and minerals play an important role in immune function and general health. They aid the body's defensive systems, boost immune cell generation and function, and help manage inflammation. A well-balanced diet rich in nutrient-dense foods is vital for acquiring sufficient amounts of these critical elements and sustaining a healthy immune system.

Chapter 3

Making an Inflammatory-Free Kitchen

The kitchen is the heart of every house, and it is also where we have the ability to make decisions that may improve our health. When it comes to inflammation management, having an anti-inflammatory kitchen might be a game changer. You may set yourself up for success in creating wholesome meals that promote your overall well-being by filling your pantry with the correct foods, having key equipment on hand, and practicing wise meal planning. Let's go through some essential procedures for making an anti-inflammatory kitchen.

Stocking Your Pantry with Anti-Inflammation Ingredients:
 Complete Grains: Choose nutrient-dense whole grains such as quinoa, brown rice, oats, and whole wheat flour. These grains are abundant in fiber and antioxidants and phytochemicals, which are anti-inflammatory components.

 Healthy Fats: Include extra virgin olive oil, avocado oil, nuts (almonds, walnuts), and seeds (chia seeds, flaxseeds) in your pantry. These lipids are high in omega-3 fatty acids and monounsaturated fats, both of which are anti-inflammatory.

 Herbs and Spices: Stock up on a range of anti-inflammatory herbs and spices, such as turmeric, ginger, cinnamon, garlic, rosemary, and oregano. These components not only add taste to your cuisine, but they also have anti-inflammatory properties.

d. Colorful Fruits and veggies: Keep fresh or frozen fruits and veggies on hand in your kitchen. Berries, leafy greens, broccoli, bell peppers, and sweet potatoes are high in antioxidants and phytochemicals that help fight inflammation.

e. Legumes: Have a variety of legumes on hand, such as lentils, chickpeas, black beans, and kidney beans. Legumes are high in plant-based protein, fiber, and antioxidants, all of which help to reduce inflammation.

f. Low-Sodium Broth and Stock: For soups and stews, use low-sodium vegetable or chicken broth. These solutions deliver taste without a lot of salt, which may cause inflammation.

g. Natural Sweeteners: Instead of refined sugar, use natural sweeteners such as honey, maple syrup, or dates. Refined sugar may cause inflammation, while natural sweeteners include more nutrients and have a smaller influence on blood sugar levels.

h. Dark Chocolate: Stock up on high-quality dark chocolate with a high cocoa content (70% or above). Anti-inflammatory antioxidants and flavonoids are found in dark chocolate.

Kitchen Tools for Simple and Healthy Cooking:
 Superior Cookware: Invest in high-quality pots, pans, and baking sheets made of stainless steel or cast iron. Nonstick cookware with a ceramic covering is also a healthy alternative.

 Sharp Knives: Keep a set of sharp knives on hand for simpler and safer cutting and slicing of veggies. Dull blades may cause ineffective cutting and increase the likelihood of an accident.

 Blender or Food Processor: A blender or food processor may be used to create smoothies, sauces, and homemade dips. It might make it easier to add nutrient-dense items into your meals.

d. Steamer Basket: Steaming is a mild cooking technique that helps veggies retain nutrients. A steamer basket enables you to swiftly and effectively steam veggies.

 Slow Cooker or Instant Pot: These devices are ideal for making nutritious soups, stews, and one-pot meals. They need less active cooking time and may aid in the tenderization of harder meats and beans.

f. Spice Grinder or Mortar and Pestle: Grinding whole spices just before using them helps to maintain their taste and strength. You may make freshly ground spices for your recipes using a spice grinder or mortar and pestle.

g. Salad Spinner: A salad spinner makes it simple to wash and dry leafy greens before using them in salads or other recipes.

 Storage Containers: Keep a range of BPA-free storage containers in various sizes on hand for storing leftovers or pre-prepared materials. Glass containers are a healthy and eco-friendly solution.

Understanding Labels: Anti-Inflammatory Product Selection: Read Ingredient Lists: When buying packaged goods, carefully study the ingredient lists. Products containing artificial additives, preservatives, hydrogenated oils, and high fructose corn syrup should be avoided since they might cause inflammation.

Look for Added Sugars: Look for added sugars in foods such as sauces, dressings, and condiments. Choose alternatives with little or no added sugars, or make your own at home.

Look for Whole Foods: Choose foods that have been minimally processed and are closer to their natural condition. Whole foods are higher in nutrients and have fewer additives that might cause inflammation.

Choose Organic: When feasible, choose organic vegetables and other items. Organic alternatives decrease exposure to pesticides and possibly hazardous substances that might cause irritation.

Convenient Meal Planning and Batch Cooking: Plan Your Meals: Spend some time each week planning your meals and making a shopping list. Incorporate a range of anti-inflammatory components into your meals to ensure nutritional balance.

Batch Cooking: Set aside a few hours each week to prepare bigger batches of specific foods. This way, you can have pre-cooked grains, roasted veggies, or a bowl of homemade soup on hand for the rest of the week.

Ingredient Steps: Wash and cut fruits and vegetables ahead of time so they're ready to use in recipes or as nutritious snacks. Preparing ingredients ahead of time saves time during meal Steps and promotes healthy eating habits.

Freezing Meals: Make extra meals and freeze them in individual servings. When you don't have time to cook from scratch, this method gives fast and simple solutions.

Making an anti-inflammatory kitchen can help you succeed in adopting an anti-inflammatory lifestyle. Stocking your pantry with nutritious products, equipping your kitchen with the necessary equipment, reading food labels, and practicing meal planning may make it simpler to cook healthy meals that promote overall health and well-being. With time and experience, your anti-inflammatory kitchen will become a haven for good behaviors and successful inflammation management.

Chapter 4

Breakfast And Brunch Recipes

Breakfast Recipes

To get you started, here are just a few breakfast suggestions. You are welcome to experiment with various ingredients and tastes to create your own scrumptious breakfast dishes. Have a great breakfast!

Scrambled Eggs with Spinach and Feta

Ingredients:

- 2 large eggs
- Handful of fresh spinach leaves
- 1/4 cup crumbled feta cheese
- Salt and pepper to taste

Steps:
- Whisk the eggs with salt and pepper in a bowl.
- Add the spinach to a nonstick skillet that is already hot over medium heat. Prepare until wilted.
- Add the beaten eggs to the pan and gently whisk while cooking them until they reach the required consistency and are scrambled.
- Feta cheese should be added before serving the scrambled eggs.

Overnight Chia Pudding

Ingredients:

- 2 tbsp chia seeds
- 1/2 cup almond milk (or any milk of your choice)
- 1 tsp honey or maple syrup
- Fresh berries or sliced fruits for topping

Steps:
- Combine the chia seeds, almond milk, and sweetener in a container or dish. Stir well.

- To help the chia seeds absorb the liquid, cover the jar or dish and place it in the refrigerator for at least 4 hours or overnight.
- Before serving, stir the mixture and top it with fresh fruit slices or berries.

Greek Yogurt Parfait

Ingredients:

- 1 cup Greek yogurt
- 1/4 cup granola
- 1/4 cup mixed berries
- 1 tbsp honey

Steps:
- Greek yogurt, granola, and mixed berries should be arranged in a glass or dish.
- Spoon honey over the top.
- Enjoy, and repeat the layers as desired.

Avocado Toast with Poached Eggs

Ingredients:

- 1 ripe avocado
- 2 slices of whole grain bread, toasted
- 2 poached eggs
- Salt, pepper, and red pepper flakes to taste

Steps:
- In a bowl, mash the avocado and add the salt, pepper, and red pepper flakes.
- Toast the bread pieces, then spread each with mashed avocado.
- Put a poached egg on top of each toast.
- If preferred, add more salt and pepper before serving.

Veggie Omelette

Ingredients:

- 3 large eggs
- 1/4 cup diced bell peppers (any color)
- 1/4 cup diced tomatoes
- 1/4 cup diced mushrooms
- 1/4 cup shredded cheddar cheese

- Salt and pepper to taste
- Fresh herbs for garnish (optional)

Steps:

The eggs should be whisked in a bowl with salt and pepper.

The bell peppers, tomatoes, and mushrooms are added to a nonstick pan that has been heated over medium heat. Cook for softening.

After adding the beaten eggs, stir the pan to ensure that they are distributed evenly over the cooked veggies.

Cheddar cheese crumbles should be sprinkled over the eggs before continuing to cook the omelette.

If preferred, top the omelette with fresh herbs before serving.

Berry Smoothie Bowl

Ingredients:

- 1 frozen banana
- 1/2 cup frozen mixed berries
- 1/2 cup almond milk (or any milk of your choice)
- Toppings: sliced banana, fresh berries, granola, chia seeds

Steps:

- Blend the frozen banana, frozen berries, and almond milk together in a blender. Blend till creamy and smooth.
- Pour the smoothie into a bowl and top with chosen ingredients, such as granola, chia seeds, sliced bananas, or fresh berries.
- Take a spoon and enjoy

Quinoa Breakfast Bowl

Ingredients:

- 1/2 cup cooked quinoa
- 1/4 cup almond milk (or any milk of your choice)
- 1 tbsp honey or maple syrup
- 1 tbsp chopped nuts (e.g., almonds, walnuts)
- 1 tbsp dried fruits (e.g., raisins, cranberries)
- Fresh fruits for topping

Steps:

- Almond milk, honey, maple syrup, chopped almonds, and dried fruit are all combined with cooked quinoa in a dish.

- Mix well, then top with your preferred fresh fruit.
- cold or warm serving.

Smoked Salmon and Cream Cheese Bagel

Ingredients:

- 1 whole wheat bagel, sliced and toasted
- 2 oz smoked salmon
- 2 tbsp cream cheese
- Sliced cucumber, red onion, and capers for topping

Steps:
- On each half of a toasted bagel, spread cream cheese.
- Add slices of smoked salmon on top.
- Sliced cucumber, red onion, and capers are used as a garnish.
- Enjoy as a sandwich or open-faced.

Coconut Banana Pancakes

Ingredients:

- 1 ripe banana, mashed
- 2 eggs
- 2 tbsp coconut flour
- 1/4 tsp baking powder
- Pinch of salt
- Coconut oil for cooking
- Fresh berries or sliced fruits for topping

Steps:
- The mashed banana and the eggs should be mixed together in a bowl.
- Salt, baking soda, and coconut flour should be added. Stir well to mix.
- In a pan over medium heat, warm coconut oil.
- On the skillet, pour approximately 1/4 cup of the pancake batter. Cook until surface bubbles appear, then turn it over and continue cooking the other side.
- Continue by using the remaining batter.

Serve the pancakes topped with sliced fruit or fresh berries.

Spinach and Mushroom Frittata

Ingredients:

- 6 large eggs

- 1 cup fresh spinach leaves
- 1/2 cup sliced mushrooms
- 1/4 cup diced onion
- 1/4 cup shredded cheese (e.g., cheddar, mozzarella)
- Salt and pepper to taste
- Fresh herbs for garnish (optional)

Steps:

- Set the oven's temperature to 350°F (175°C).
- Sauté the onions and mushrooms in an oven-safe pan until they are tender.
- Spinach leaves should be added and cooked until wilted.
- Whisk the eggs with the cheese shredded, salt, and pepper in a bowl.
- Over the skillet's sautéed veggies, pour the egg mixture.
- Cook on the stovetop for a few minutes over medium heat, or until the edges begin to firm.
- Bake the frittata for approximately 15 minutes, or until it is set and just beginning to turn brown, in the preheated oven.
- If preferred, garnish with fresh herbs before serving.

Peanut Butter Banana Toast

Ingredients:

- 2 slices of whole grain bread, toasted
- 2 tbsp peanut butter
- 1 ripe banana, sliced
- Honey or maple syrup for drizzling (optional)

Steps:

- On each piece of bread, evenly spread peanut butter.
- Place banana slices on top.
- If desired, drizzle with honey or maple syrup.
- Eat it like a conventional sandwich or an open-faced sandwich.

Baked Egg Cups

Ingredients:

- 6 large eggs
- 1/4 cup diced bell peppers (any color)
- 1/4 cup diced tomatoes
- 1/4 cup diced ham or cooked bacon
- Salt and pepper to taste
- Chopped fresh herbs for garnish (optional)

Steps:

- Set the oven's temperature to 350°F (175°C).
- A muffin pan should be greased or lined with silicone muffin liners.
- Whisk the eggs with salt and pepper in a bowl.
- Distribute equally among the muffin cups the diced tomatoes, ham or bacon, and bell peppers.
- Over the contents in each cup, pour the beaten eggs.
- Bake for 15 to 18 minutes, or until the eggs are set, in the preheated oven.
- Remove from the oven, let it cool slightly, and then, if you want, garnish with fresh herbs before serving.

Fruit and Yogurt Parfait

Ingredients:

- 1 cup Greek yogurt
- 1/4 cup granola
- Assorted fresh fruits (e.g., berries, sliced peaches, kiwi)
- Honey or maple syrup for drizzling (optional)

Steps:

- Greek yogurt, granola, and fresh fruit should be arranged in a glass or dish.
- If desired, drizzle with honey or maple syrup.
- If desired, repeat the layers. Enjoy.

Mexican Breakfast Burrito

Ingredients:

- 2 large eggs, beaten
- 2 small whole wheat tortillas
- 1/4 cup black beans, drained and rinsed
- 2 tbsp salsa
- 2 tbsp shredded cheese (e.g., cheddar, Monterey Jack)
- Chopped fresh cilantro for garnish (optional)

Steps:

- The beaten eggs should be fried in a pan over medium heat.
- The tortillas should be warmed briefly in the microwave or a dry skillet.
- In the middle of each tortilla, distribute half of the scrambled eggs.
- Add salsa, shredded cheese, chopped cilantro, and black beans as garnish.
- The tortilla's sides should be folded toward the center before being securely rolled.
- If preferred, cut the tortilla in half before serving.

Blueberry Oatmeal

Ingredients:

- 1/2 cup rolled oats
- 1 cup water or milk (dairy or plant-based)
- 1/4 cup fresh or frozen blueberries
- 1 tbsp honey or maple syrup
- Chopped nuts or seeds for topping (e.g., almonds, walnuts, chia seeds)

Steps:

- Bring milk or water to a boil in a saucepan.
- Turn the heat down to medium-low after adding the rolled oats.
- The oats should be creamy and soft after approximately 5 minutes of cooking and sporadically tossing.
- The blueberries should be heated through after being added, so stir them in.
- Honey or maple syrup should be added after the mixture has been taken off the heat.
- Add chopped nuts or seeds to the oats in a bowl before serving.

Breakfast Quinoa Bowl

Ingredients:

- 1/2 cup cooked quinoa
- 1/4 cup almond milk (or any milk of your choice)
- 1 tbsp honey or maple syrup
- 1/4 cup mixed nuts and seeds (e.g., almonds, walnuts, pumpkin seeds)
- Fresh fruits for topping

Steps:

- Cooked quinoa, almond milk, honey or maple syrup, and a variety of nuts and seeds should all be combined in a dish.
- Mix well, then top with your preferred fresh fruit.
- You may serve it hot or cold.

Ham and Cheese Breakfast Wrap

Ingredients:

- 1 large whole wheat tortilla
- 2 slices of ham
- 2 slices of cheese (e.g., Swiss, cheddar)
- Sliced tomatoes and lettuce for topping
- Mustard or mayonnaise (optional)

Steps:

- The ham and cheese slices should be placed on one side of the flattened tortill
- Add lettuce and tomato slices on top.
- If desired, include mustard or mayonnaise.
- The tortilla's sides should be folded toward the center before being securely rolled.
- If preferred, cut the wrap in half before serving.

Apple Cinnamon Overnight Oats

Ingredients:

- 1/2 cup rolled oats
- 1/2 cup almond milk (or any milk of your choice)
- 1/4 cup unsweetened applesauce
- 1 tbsp honey or maple syrup
- 1/4 tsp cinnamon
- Chopped apples and walnuts for topping

Steps:

- Rolling oats, almond milk, applesauce, honey or maple syrup, and cinnamon should all be combined in a container or dish. Stir well.
- To help the oats soften and absorb the liquid, cover the jar or dish and place it in the refrigerator for at least 4 hours or overnight.
- Before serving, give the mixture a stir and sprinkle chopped apples and walnuts over top.

Vegetable and Cheese Omelette

Ingredients:

- 3 large eggs
- 1/4 cup diced bell peppers (any color)
- 1/4 cup diced zucchini
- 1/4 cup diced onion
- 1/4 cup shredded cheese (e.g., mozzarella, feta)
- Salt and pepper to taste
- Fresh herbs for garnish (optional)

Steps:

- The eggs should be beaten with salt and pepper in a basin.
- The bell peppers, zucchini, and onion are added to a nonstick pan that has been heated over medium heat. Cook for softening.

- After adding the beaten eggs, stir the pan to ensure that they are distributed evenly over the cooked veggies.
- Once the omelette is ready, sprinkle the cheese shreds over the eggs.
- If preferred, top the omelette with fresh herbs before serving.

Breakfast Quesadilla

Ingredients:

- 2 small whole wheat tortillas
- 2 eggs, scrambled
- 2 slices of cooked bacon, crumbled
- 2 tbsp shredded cheese (e.g., cheddar, Monterey Jack)
- Sliced avocado and salsa for topping

Steps:
- The eggs should be prepared by scrambling them in a pan over medium heat.
- Spread scrambled eggs, crumbled bacon, and shredded cheese equally over one tortilla that has been laid out flat.
- For a quesadilla, place the second tortilla on top.
- When the tortillas are crisp and the cheese is melted, cook the quesadilla in a pan over medium heat, turning once.
- Sliced avocado and salsa should be served with the dish once it is removed from the heat.

Green Smoothie

Ingredients:

- 1 ripe banana
- 1 cup fresh spinach leaves
- 1/2 cup almond milk (or any milk of your choice)
- 1/2 cup Greek yogurt
- 1 tbsp honey or maple syrup

Steps:
- Blend the ripe banana with the spinach leaves, Greek yogurt, honey, or maple syrup in a blender.
- Blend till creamy and smooth.
- Place in a glass and sip.

Sausage and Veggie Breakfast Skillet

Ingredients:

- 2 sausages, sliced

- 1/2 cup diced bell peppers (any color)
- 1/2 cup diced zucchini
- 1/4 cup diced onion
- Salt, pepper, and paprika to taste
- 2 eggs

Steps:

- The sliced sausages should be cooked thoroughly and browned in a pan over medium heat.
- To the pan, add the onion, bell pepper, and zucchini that have been diced. Cook the veggies until they are tender.
- To taste, add paprika, salt, and pepper.
- In the skillet, make two wells and break one egg into each of them.
- Cook the eggs in the covered skillet until they reach the desired doneness.
- Breakfast on a pan should be hot.

Cinnamon French Toast

Ingredients:

- 2 slices of whole wheat bread
- 2 large eggs
- 1/4 cup milk (dairy or plant-based)
- 1/2 tsp vanilla extract
- 1/2 tsp cinnamon
- Maple syrup and fresh fruits for topping

Steps:

- Whisk the eggs, milk, vanilla extract, and cinnamon in a small basin.
- Make sure both sides of each piece of bread are covered by dipping it into the egg mixture.
- Cooking spray or butter may be used to gently oil a non-stick pan or griddle.
- Slices of dipping bread should be placed in the pan and cooked until both sides are golden brown.
- With fresh fruits on top, remove from the heat and sprinkle with maple syrup.

Protein-Packed Breakfast Burrito

Ingredients:

- 2 large eggs, beaten
- 1/4 cup black beans, drained and rinsed
- 1/4 cup diced tomatoes
- 2 tbsp diced red onion
- 2 tbsp shredded cheese (e.g., cheddar, pepper jack)
- 2 whole wheat tortillas
- Salsa and sliced avocado for topping

Steps:

- The beaten eggs should be fried in a pan over medium heat.
- To the pan, add the diced red onion, diced tomatoes, and black beans. Stir constantly until fully warmed.
- The tortillas should be warmed briefly in the microwave or a dry skillet.
- Between the tortillas, distribute the scrambled egg mixture and the cheese.
- Avocado slices and salsa are added on top.
- The tortilla's sides should be folded toward the center before being securely rolled.
- If preferred, cut the tortilla in half before serving.

Raspberry Almond Chia Pudding

Ingredients:

- 2 tbsp chia seeds
- 1/2 cup almond milk (or any milk of your choice)
- 1/4 cup fresh or frozen raspberries
- 1 tbsp honey or maple syrup
- Sliced almonds and additional raspberries for topping

Steps:

- Chia seeds and almond milk are combined in a container or dish. Stir well.
- Add honey or maple syrup, as well as fresh or frozen raspberries. Again, stir.
- To enable the chia seeds to thicken, cover the jar or dish and place it in the refrigerator for at least 2 hours or overnight.
- Before serving, stir the mixture, then sprinkle more raspberries and sliced almonds on top.

Avocado Toast with Egg

Ingredients:

- 2 slices of whole grain bread, toasted

- 1 ripe avocado, mashed
- 2 eggs, cooked to your preference (e.g., fried, poached, scrambled)
- Salt, pepper, and red pepper flakes to taste
- Fresh herbs for garnish (e.g., cilantro, parsley)

Steps:

- On each toast, equally distribute the mashed avocado.
- Add a fried egg on top.
- To taste, add salt, pepper, and red pepper flakes.
- Serve with fresh herbs as a garnish.

Banana Nut Overnight Oats

Ingredients:

- 1/2 cup rolled oats
- 1/2 cup almond milk (or any milk of your choice)
- 1 ripe banana, mashed
- 1 tbsp honey or maple syrup
- 1 tbsp chopped nuts (e.g., walnuts, almonds)
- Dash of cinnamon

Steps:

- Rollin oats, almond milk, mashed banana, honey or maple syrup, chopped almonds, and cinnamon should all be combined in a jar or other container. Stir well.
- To help the oats soften and absorb the liquid, cover the jar or container and place it in the refrigerator for at least 4 hours or overnight.
- Before serving, stir the ingredients, then serve cold.

Veggie Breakfast Wrap

Ingredients:

- 1 large whole wheat tortilla
- 2 eggs, scrambled
- 1/4 cup diced bell peppers (any color)
- 1/4 cup diced tomatoes
- 2 tbsp diced red onion
- Sliced avocado and fresh spinach leaves for topping

Steps:

- In a skillet, scramble the eggs over medium heat until cooked.
- Add the diced bell peppers, tomatoes, and red onion to the skillet. Cook until the vegetables are softened.
- Warm the tortilla in a dry skillet or microwave for a few seconds.

- Place the scrambled egg mixture onto the tortilla.
- Top with sliced avocado and fresh spinach leaves.
- Fold the sides of the tortilla toward the center, then roll it up tightly.
- Slice the wrap in half if desired and serve.

Mediterranean Egg Muffins

Ingredients:

- 6 large eggs
- 1/4 cup diced red bell pepper
- 1/4 cup diced red onion
- 1/4 cup diced tomatoes
- 1/4 cup crumbled feta cheese
- 1 tbsp chopped fresh parsley
- Salt and pepper to taste

Steps:

- As soon as the oven reaches 350°F (175°C), oil or line a muffin pan with silicone muffin cups.
- Whisk the eggs with salt and pepper in a bowl.
- Distribute equally among the muffin cups the diced red bell pepper, red onion, tomatoes, feta cheese, and parsley.
- Each cup should be filled approximately 3/4 full with the beaten eggs before being placed on a plate.
- Bake for 18 to 20 minutes, or until the eggs are set, in the preheated oven.
- Take out of the oven, let it cool a little, and then serve.

Peanut Butter and Jelly Smoothie

Ingredients:

- 1 ripe banana
- 1 cup almond milk (or any milk of your choice)
- 2 tbsp peanut butter
- 1 tbsp jelly (any flavor)
- 1/2 cup ice cubes

Steps:

- Put the ripe banana, almond milk, peanut butter, jelly, and ice cubes in a blender.
- Blend till creamy and smooth.
- Place in a glass and sip.

Brunch Recipes

Avocado Toast with Poached Eggs:

Ingredients:

- 2 slices of whole grain bread
- 1 ripe avocado
- 2 eggs
- Salt and pepper to taste
- Optional toppings: red pepper flakes, chopped fresh herbs

steps:

- Bread pieces should be toasted till golden brown.
- Slice the avocado in half, scrape out the pit, and place the avocado flesh in a bowl. With a fork, mash the avocado until it is smooth.
- To poach the eggs, add water to a medium pot and bring it to a low simmer. In separate little dishes or ramekins, crack the eggs. The eggs should be delicately lowered into the middle of the boiling water to create a moderate vortex. For a soft, runny yolk, cook for 3–4 minutes. For a firmer yolk, cook for longer.
- Each piece of toast should have a uniform layer of mashed avocado. Add salt and pepper to taste.
- With a slotted spoon, carefully take the poached eggs from the water, and then arrange one over each piece of avocado toast.

If desired, top with more toppings. Serve right away.

Berry and Yogurt Parfait:

Ingredients:

- 1 cup Greek yogurt
- 1 cup mixed berries (strawberries, blueberries, raspberries)
- ¼ cup granola
- 1 tablespoon honey
- Optional toppings: chopped nuts, shredded coconut

steps:

- Layer half of the Greek yogurt in a glass or container.
- On top of the yogurt, sprinkle half of the mixed berries

- Over the berries, scatter the other half of the granola.
- Over the granola, drizzle half of the honey.
- With the remaining ingredients, repeat the stacking procedure.
- Add optional toppings to complete, if desired.

Either serve right now or store in the fridge.

Vegetable Frittata:

Ingredients:

- 6 eggs
- ½ cup milk
- 1 cup chopped mixed vegetables (bell peppers, onions, spinach, mushrooms, etc.)
- ½ cup shredded cheese (cheddar, mozzarella, or your choice)
- Salt and pepper to taste
- 1 tablespoon olive oil

Steps

- Set the oven's temperature to 375°F (190°C).
- Combine the milk and eggs in a bowl. Add salt and pepper to taste.
- In a pan that may be used in the oven, warm the olive oil. The veggies should be sautéed after being chopped.
- Over the skillet's sautéed veggies, pour the egg mixture. To spread the veggies evenly, gently stir.
- On top, scatter the cheese shavings.
- Bake the frittata for approximately 15-20 minutes, or until it is set and brown on top, in the preheated oven.
- Before slicing, take it out of the oven and let it cool somewhat.
- Serve either warm or at room temperature.

Smoked Salmon Bagel:

Ingredients:

- 1 bagel, sliced in half
- 2-3 ounces smoked salmon
- 2 tablespoons cream cheese
- Sliced red onion

- Capers
- Fresh dill

Steps
- Bagel halves should be gently toasted till browned.
- On each half of the bagel, spread cream cheese.
- Cream cheese is layered on top of smoked salmon.
- Red onion slices and capers should also be included.
- Add some fresh dill as garnish.
- Serve right away.

Spinach and Mushroom Quiche:

Ingredients:

- 1 pre-made pie crust
- 4 eggs
- ½ cup milk
- 1 cup fresh spinach, chopped
- ½ cup mushrooms, sliced
- ½ cup shredded cheese (Gruyere, Swiss, or your choice)
- Salt and pepper to taste
- 1 tablespoon olive oil

Steps
- Set the oven's temperature to 375°F (190°C).
- Set aside the pie crust in a pie plate.
- In a pan over medium heat, warm the olive oil. Add the mushrooms and cook them for a few minutes, or until they give off moisture and become golden brown. Add the spinach and cook it until it wilts. Get rid of the heat.
- Combine the milk and eggs in a bowl. Add salt and pepper to taste.
- Over the bottom of the pie crust, evenly distribute the sautéed veggies.
- Over the veggies, pour the egg mixture.
- On top, scatter the cheese shavings.
- Bake the quiche in a preheated oven for 30-35 minutes, or until the filling is set and the crust is brown.
- Before slicing, take it out of the oven and let it cool somewhat.
- At room temperature or heated, serve.

Banana Pancakes:

Ingredients:

- 1 cup all-purpose flour
- 1 tablespoon sugar
- 1 teaspoon baking powder
- ½ teaspoon baking soda
- Pinch of salt
- 1 ripe banana, mashed
- 1 cup buttermilk
- 1 large egg
- 2 tablespoons melted butter
- Optional toppings: sliced bananas, maple syrup, chopped nuts

Steps

- Combine the flour, sugar, baking soda, baking powder, and salt in a mixing dish.
- Whisk the mashed banana, buttermilk, egg, and melted butter in another basin.
- After adding the liquid components, mix the dry ingredients just until they are barely blended. Avoid overmixing; a few lumps are OK.
- Butter or frying spray should be used to gently oil a non-stick pan or griddle before heating it up.
- For each pancake, add roughly 14 cups of the pancake batter to the skillet.
- Cook until surface bubbles appear, turn, and cook for an additional 1 to 2 minutes, or until golden brown.
- Continue by using the remaining batter.
- Warm banana pancakes may be served with extra toppings.

Quinoa Breakfast Bowl:

Ingredients:

- 1 cup cooked quinoa
- ½ cup Greek yogurt
- ½ cup mixed berries
- 2 tablespoons honey or maple syrup
- 2 tablespoons chopped nuts (almonds, walnuts, etc.)
- Optional toppings: chia seeds, coconut flakes, sliced bananas

Steps

- Greek yogurt and cooked quinoa should be combined in a dish.

- Add some mixed berries on top and finish with some honey or maple syrup.
- If desired, top with extra toppings and chopped nuts.
- The quinoa breakfast dish should be served right away.

Vegetable and Goat Cheese Omelette:

Ingredients:

- 3 eggs
- 2 tablespoons milk
- ½ cup chopped mixed vegetables (bell peppers, onions, zucchini, etc.)
- 2 tablespoons crumbled goat cheese
- Salt and pepper to taste
- 1 tablespoon olive oil or butter

Steps
- Whisk the eggs, milk, salt, and pepper in a bowl.
- In a non-stick skillet, heat butter or olive oil over medium heat.
- The vegetables should be sautéed after being chopped.
- In order to spread the eggs evenly, pour the egg mixture into the skillet while tilting it.
- Cook the omelette just until the edges begin to firm.
- Over one half of the omelette, scatter the goat cheese that has been crushed.
- Over the cheese, gently fold the other half of the omelette.
- Cook the omelette for one more minute, or until the cheese has melted and it is thoroughly cooked.
- Place the hot omelette on a dish after sliding it there.

Blueberry Muffins:

Ingredients:

- 1 ½ cups all-purpose flour
- ½ cup sugar
- 2 teaspoons baking powder
- ½ teaspoon salt
- 1/3 cup melted butter
- ½ cup milk
- 1 large egg
- 1 teaspoon vanilla extract
- 1 cup fresh or frozen blueberries

Steps

- Set the oven's temperature to 375°F (190°C). Use paper liners or butter the cups of a muffin pan.
- Combine the flour, sugar, baking soda, and salt in a sizable mixing bowl.
- Whisk the melted butter, milk, egg, and vanilla extract in a separate basin.
- After adding the liquid components, mix the dry ingredients only until they are barely blended.
- Fold the blueberries in slowly.
- Fill each muffin cup about two-thirds full after dividing the batter equally among them.
- 18 to 20 minutes of baking time, or until a toothpick inserted in the center of the cake comes out clean.
- After removing the muffins from the oven, let them cool in the pan for a short while before moving them to a wire rack to finish cooling.
- The blueberry muffins should be served at room temperature.

Huevos Rancheros:

Ingredients:

- 2 corn tortillas
- 2 eggs
- ½ cup black beans, drained and rinsed
- ¼ cup salsa
- 2 tablespoons chopped fresh cilantro
- Salt and pepper to taste
- Optional toppings: sliced avocado, crumbled feta cheese, sour cream

Steps

- The corn tortillas should be warmed in a nonstick skillet over medium heat until they are flexible.
- Fry the eggs to the desired doneness in the same skillet.
- In the meantime, warm the black beans completely in a small pot.
- To assemble, spread half of the warmed black beans on a platter and top with a tortilla.
- Fry an egg and place it on top of the beans.
- Add salsa and cilantro sprigs to the top of the egg.
- Add salt and pepper to taste.
- The remaining tortilla, beans, egg, salsa, and cilantro should be used in the same manner.

- Add extra garnishes if you would like.
- Warm the eggs rancheros before serving.

French Toast with Mixed Berries:

Ingredients:

- 4 slices of bread (white, whole grain, or your choice)
- 2 eggs
- ¼ cup milk
- 1 teaspoon vanilla extract
- 1 tablespoon butter
- 1 cup mixed berries
- Powdered sugar for dusting
- Maple syrup for serving

Steps
- Whisk the eggs, milk, and vanilla extract in a shallow dish.
- In a nonstick skillet, melt butter over medium heat.
- Each piece of bread should be dipped into the egg mixture and given a quick soak on both sides.
- In the skillet, add the moistened bread, and cook for two to three minutes per side, or until golden brown.
- French toast should be taken out of the skillet and kept warm.
- The mixed berries should be heated thoroughly and slightly cooked in the same skillet.
- Place the warm mixed berries on top of the French toast on plates and sprinkle with powdered sugar.
- Add maple syrup to the dish.

Greek Yogurt Pancakes:

Ingredients:

- 1 cup all-purpose flour
- 2 tablespoons sugar
- 1 teaspoon baking powder
- ½ teaspoon baking soda
- Pinch of salt
- 1 cup Greek yogurt
- ½ cup milk

- 1 large egg
- 1 teaspoon vanilla extract
- Optional toppings: sliced fresh fruit, honey, Greek yogurt

Steps
- Combine the flour, sugar, baking soda, baking powder, and salt in a mixing dish.
- Whisk the Greek yogurt, milk, egg, and vanilla extract in another bowl.
- After adding the liquid components, mix the dry ingredients only until they are barely blended. Avoid overmixing; a few lumps are acceptable.
- Butter or frying spray should be used to lightly oil a non-stick pan or griddle before heating it up.
- For each pancake, add roughly 14 cups of the pancake batter to the skillet.
- Cook until surface bubbles appear, flip, and cook for an additional 1 to 2 minutes, or until golden brown.
- Continue by using the remaining batter.
- Warm Greek yogurt pancakes can be topped with other ingredients.

Sausage and Spinach Breakfast Wrap:

Ingredients:

- 4 large eggs
- 2 tablespoons milk
- Salt and pepper to taste
- 4 large whole wheat tortillas
- 4 cooked breakfast sausage links, sliced
- 1 cup fresh spinach leaves
- ½ cup shredded cheese (cheddar, mozzarella, or your choice)

Steps
- Whisk the eggs, milk, salt, and pepper in a bowl.
- Scramble the eggs in a nonstick skillet over medium heat until they are done to your taste.
- The whole wheat tortillas can be warmed in a microwave or a dry skillet.
- The scrambled eggs, sliced sausage, spinach leaves, and shredded cheese should be arranged on top of a tortilla on a level surface.
- The tortilla should be securely rolled, tucking in the sides as you go.
- With the remaining tortillas and filling ingredients, repeat the procedure.
- Breakfast wraps with sausage and spinach should be served hot.

Veggie Breakfast Burrito:

Ingredients:

- 4 large eggs
- 2 tablespoons milk
- Salt and pepper to taste
- 4 large whole wheat tortillas
- ½ cup black beans, drained and rinsed
- ½ cup chopped mixed vegetables (bell peppers, onions, zucchini, etc.)
- ½ cup shredded cheese (cheddar, mozzarella, or your choice)
- Optional toppings: salsa, avocado slices, sour cream

Steps

- Whisk the eggs, milk, salt, and pepper in a bowl.
- Scramble the eggs in a nonstick skillet over medium heat until they are done to your taste.
- The whole wheat tortillas can be warmed in a microwave or a dry skillet.
- Scrambled eggs, black beans, finely chopped veggies, and shredded cheese should be spread out on a flat surface.
- The tortilla should be securely rolled, tucking in the sides as you go.
- With the remaining tortillas and filling ingredients, repeat the procedure.
- Add more garnishes if you'd like.
- Warm the breakfast burritos with vegetables.

Breakfast Quinoa Bowl:

Ingredients:

- 1 cup cooked quinoa
- ½ cup Greek yogurt
- ¼ cup mixed nuts and seeds (almonds, walnuts, pumpkin seeds, etc.)
- 2 tablespoons dried cranberries or raisins
- 1 tablespoon honey or maple syrup
- Optional toppings: sliced fresh fruit, coconut flakes, cinnamon

Steps

- Greek yogurt and cooked quinoa should be combined in a bowl.
- Add dried cranberries, raisins, or mixed nuts and seeds on top, then drizzle with honey or maple syrup.
- Add more garnishes if you'd like.

- The breakfast quinoa bowl should be served right away.

Breakfast BLT:

Ingredients:

- 4 slices of bread (white, whole grain, or your choice)
- 4 slices of cooked bacon
- 2 large lettuce leaves
- 1 ripe tomato, sliced
- Mayonnaise

steps
- Bread pieces should be lightly toasted till golden.
- Each slice should have mayonnaise spread on one side.
- On two slices of bread, arrange the tomato, lettuce, and bacon.
- Add the remaining bread slices on top, mayo side down.
- Cut the sandwiches in half diagonally.
- Serve the BLTs for breakfast right away.

Hash Brown Casserole:

Ingredients:

- 4 cups frozen shredded hash browns, thawed
- 1 cup shredded cheddar cheese
- ½ cup sour cream
- ½ cup milk
- 4 green onions, chopped
- Salt and pepper to taste
- Optional toppings: chopped fresh parsley, diced tomatoes

Steps
- Set the oven's temperature to 375°F (190°C). Butter a baking pan.
- Hash browns that have been thawed, shredded cheddar cheese, sour cream, milk, finely chopped green onions, salt, and pepper should all be combined in a big bowl. Mix thoroughly.
- Spread out the mixture evenly in the prepared baking dish after transfer.
- Bake the hash browns for 30-35 minutes, or until the tops are crispy and golden.
- Before serving, take it out of the oven and allow it cool somewhat.

- If desired, top with more toppings.
- Hash brown casserole should be served hot.

Pancetta and Mushroom Quiche:

Ingredients:

- 1 pre-made pie crust
- 4 eggs
- ½ cup milk
- 1 cup sliced mushrooms
- ¼ cup cooked pancetta, chopped
- ½ cup shredded cheese (Gruyere, Swiss, or your choice)
- Salt and pepper to taste
- 1 tablespoon olive oil

Steps
- Set the oven's temperature to 375°F (190°C).
- Set aside the pie crust in a pie plate.
- In a skillet over medium heat, warm the olive oil. Sliced mushrooms should be added and sautéed until they release moisture and turn golden brown. Stir for another minute after adding the cooked pancetta. Get rid of the heat.
- Combine the milk and eggs in a bowl. Add salt and pepper to taste.
- Over the bottom of the pie crust, evenly distribute the pancetta and sautéed mushrooms.
- Over the pancetta and mushrooms, pour the egg mixture.
- On top, scatter the cheese shavings.
- Bake the quiche in a preheated oven for 30-35 minutes, or until the filling is set and the crust is brown.
- Before slicing, take it out of the oven and let it cool somewhat.
- Warm or room temperature pancetta and mushroom quiche is appropriate for serving.

Spinach and Feta Breakfast Wrap:

Ingredients:

- 4 large eggs
- 2 tablespoons milk
- Salt and pepper to taste

- 4 large whole wheat tortillas
- 1 cup fresh spinach leaves
- ½ cup crumbled feta cheese
- Optional toppings: sliced cherry tomatoes, kalamata olives, tzatziki sauce

Steps
- Whisk the eggs, milk, salt, and pepper in a bowl.
- Scramble the eggs in a nonstick skillet over medium heat until they are done to your taste.
- The whole wheat tortillas can be warmed in a microwave or a dry skillet.
- Scrambled eggs, fresh spinach, and feta cheese crumbles should be arranged on top of a tortilla on a flat surface.
- The tortilla should be securely rolled, tucking in the sides as you go.
- With the remaining tortillas and filling ingredients, repeat the procedure.
- Add more garnishes if you'd like.
- Serve the breakfast wraps with spinach and feta warm.

Greek Yogurt Parfait:

Ingredients:
- 1 cup Greek yogurt
- ¼ cup granola
- ½ cup mixed berries
- 1 tablespoon honey
- Optional toppings: sliced almonds, shredded coconut

Steps
- Greek yogurt, granola, mixed berries, and honey should be arranged in a glass or bowl.
- Continue adding layers.
- If desired, top with more toppings.
- The Greek yogurt parfait should be served right away.

Breakfast Quesadilla:

Ingredients:

- 2 large flour tortillas
- 2 large eggs, scrambled
- ½ cup shredded cheese (cheddar, Monterey Jack, or your choice)
- ¼ cup diced bell peppers
- 2 tablespoons chopped fresh cilantro

- Salt and pepper to taste
- Optional toppings: salsa, sour cream, guacamole

Steps

- A nonstick skillet should be heated to medium.
- One tortilla should be placed in the skillet along with half of the shredded cheese.
- Over the cheese, distribute the scrambled eggs, diced
- bell peppers, and chopped cilantro.
- Add salt and pepper to taste.
- Gently press down on the second tortilla after placing it on top.
- The bottom tortilla should be golden brown after a few minutes of cooking. Carefully flip the quesadilla over and continue cooking until the second tortilla is golden brown and the cheese has melted.
- Slice into wedges after removing from the skillet and let it cool for a moment.
- Warm breakfast quesadillas can be served with extra toppings.

Apple Cinnamon Oatmeal:

Ingredients:

- 1 cup rolled oats
- 2 cups water
- 1 apple, peeled, cored, and diced
- 2 tablespoons honey or maple syrup
- ½ teaspoon cinnamon
- Pinch of salt
- Optional toppings: chopped nuts, dried cranberries, yogurt

Steps

- Bring the water to a boil in a saucepan.
- Add the salt, cinnamon, honey or maple syrup, diced apple, and rolled oats.
- Stir thoroughly and turn the heat down to low.
- Stirring regularly, simmer for about 5 minutes or until the oats are mushy and the apple is soft.
- After taking it off the heat, wait a minute.
- Warm apple cinnamon oatmeal with optional toppings is served.

Spinach and Mushroom Frittata:

Ingredients:

- 6 large eggs
- ½ cup milk
- Salt and pepper to taste
- 1 tablespoon olive oil
- 1 cup sliced mushrooms
- 2 cups fresh spinach leaves
- ¼ cup shredded cheese (cheddar, Swiss, or your choice)

Steps

- Set the oven's temperature to 350°F (175°C).
- Whisk the eggs, milk, salt, and pepper in a bowl.
- In a skillet that may be used in the oven, warm the olive oil.
- Sliced mushrooms should be added and sautéed until they release moisture and turn golden brown.
- Fresh spinach leaves should be added and sautéed until wilted.
- On top of the spinach and mushrooms, pour the egg mixture.
- On top, scatter the cheese shavings.
- When the frittata is set and the cheese is melted and brown, place the pan in the preheated oven and bake for about 15-20 minutes.
- Before slicing, take it out of the oven and let it cool somewhat.
- The spinach and mushroom frittata can be served hot or cold.

Greek Spinach and Feta Omelette:

Ingredients:

- 4 large eggs
- 2 tablespoons milk
- Salt and pepper to taste
- 1 tablespoon olive oil
- 1 cup fresh spinach leaves
- ¼ cup crumbled feta cheese
- 2 tablespoons chopped fresh dill

Steps

- Whisk the eggs, milk, salt, and pepper in a bowl.
- In a non-stick skillet, warm up the olive oil over medium heat.
- Fresh spinach leaves should be added and sautéed until wilted.

- The edges should solidify after one minute of untouched cooking after pouring the egg mixture into the skillet.
- Over one side of the omelette, top with the feta cheese crumbles and fresh dill cut into small pieces.
- Fold the remaining omelette in half gently over the contents.
- Cook the omelette for one more minute, or until the cheese has melted and it is thoroughly cooked.
- Before slicing, slide the omelette onto a platter to cool for a moment.
- The Greek spinach and feta omelette should be served hot.

Chia Pudding:

Ingredients:

- 1 cup milk (dairy or plant-based)
- 3 tablespoons chia seeds
- 1 tablespoon honey or maple syrup
- ½ teaspoon vanilla extract
- Optional toppings: fresh berries, sliced banana, chopped nuts

Steps
- Combine the milk, chia seeds, honey (or maple syrup), and vanilla essence in a container or bowl.
- To make sure the chia seeds are completely submerged in the liquid, stir thoroughly.
- Give the mixture another swirl to break up any chia seed clumps after letting it settle for about 5 minutes.
- To enable the chia seeds to absorb the liquid and thicken into a pudding-like consistency, cover the jar or bowl and place in the refrigerator for at least 2 hours or overnight.
- Before serving, give the chia pudding a stir and sprinkle with any preferred toppings.
- Chia pudding should be served chilled.

Enjoy these delectable recipes for brunch!

Chapter 5

Nourishing Lunch and Dinner Recipes

Lunch Recipes

Quinoa Salad with Roasted Vegetables

Ingredients:

- 1 cup quinoa
- Assorted vegetables (such as bell peppers, zucchini, and cherry tomatoes)
- Olive oil
- Salt and pepper
- Fresh herbs (such as basil or parsley)
- Lemon juice

Steps

- Quinoa should be prepared as directed on the package and then let to cool.
- Set the oven's temperature to 400°F (200°C).
- Spread the vegetables out on a baking sheet after tossing them with olive oil, salt, and pepper.
- The veggies should be roasted in the oven for around 20 minutes, or until they are soft and just browned.
- The cooked quinoa, roasted veggies, fresh herbs, and a squeeze of lemon juice should all be combined in a big bowl. Mix well, then plate.

Spinach and Feta Stuffed Chicken Breast

Ingredients:

- Chicken breast
- Fresh spinach leaves
- Feta cheese
- Garlic powder
- Salt and pepper
- Olive oil

Steps

- Set the oven's temperature to 375°F (190°C).

- Make a pocket in the chicken breast without going through completely.
- Fill the pocket with feta cheese crumbles and spinach leaves.
- Salt, pepper, and garlic powder are used to season the chicken breast.
- In a skillet that is oven-safe, heat the olive oil over medium-high heat.
- For two to three minutes on each side, brown the chicken breast in the pan.
- Bake the skillet in the oven for 15 to 20 minutes, or until the chicken is thoroughly done.

Lentil Soup

Ingredients:

- 1 cup dried lentils
- Onion, chopped
- Carrots, diced
- Celery, diced
- Garlic, minced
- Vegetable or chicken broth
- Cumin
- Paprika
- Salt and pepper
- Fresh parsley, chopped

Steps

- Lentils should be rinsed in cold water.
- The onion, carrots, celery, and garlic should be sautéed till tender in a big pot.
- In the pot, combine the lentils, broth, cumin, paprika, salt, and pepper.
- When the lentils are ready, turn down the heat and let the stew simmer for 30 to 40 minutes.
- Before serving, add fresh parsley as a garnish and taste the spice.

Greek Salad with Grilled Chicken

Ingredients:

- Grilled chicken breast, sliced
- Romaine lettuce, chopped
- Cucumber, diced
- Cherry tomatoes, halved
- Kalamata olives
- Red onion, thinly sliced
- Feta cheese, crumbled
- Lemon juice

- Extra virgin olive oil
- Dried oregano
- Salt and pepper

Steps

- Toss together the lettuce, cucumber, tomatoes, olives, and red onion in a large salad dish.
- Sliced grilled chicken breast should be added to the salad.
- To make the dressing, combine the lemon juice, olive oil, dried oregano, salt, and pepper in a small bowl.
- Over the salad, drizzle the dressing, and mix to blend.
- Before serving, top with feta cheese crumbles.

Sweet Potato and Black Bean Tacos

Ingredients:

- Sweet potatoes, peeled and diced
- Black beans, cooked and drained
- Red bell pepper, diced
- Red onion, diced
- Garlic, minced
- Ground cumin
- Smoked paprika
- Chili powder
- Salt and pepper
- Corn tortillas
- Avocado slices
- Fresh cilantro, chopped

Steps

- Set the oven's temperature to 400°F (200°C).
- Toss the diced red bell pepper, red onion, garlic, black beans, cumin, paprika, and chili powder with the olive oil. Season with salt, pepper, and a few more spices.
- Spread the mixture on a baking sheet, then bake the sweet potatoes for 25 to 30 minutes, or until they are soft but still slightly crisp.
- Corn tortillas should be warmed up in a dry skillet over medium heat.
- The mixture of roasted sweet potatoes and black beans should be put inside the tortillas.
- Add fresh cilantro and slices of avocado on top.

Mediterranean Quinoa Bowl

Ingredients:

- Cooked quinoa
- Chickpeas, drained and rinsed
- Cucumber, diced
- Cherry tomatoes, halved
- Kalamata olives
- Red onion, thinly sliced
- Fresh parsley, chopped
- Lemon juice
- Extra virgin olive oil
- Salt and pepper
- Optional: crumbled feta cheese

Steps

- Chickpeas, cucumber, tomatoes, olives, red onion, fresh parsley, and cooked quinoa should all be combined in a bowl.
- To create the dressing, combine the lemon juice, olive oil, salt, and pepper in a small bowl.
- Over the quinoa bowl, drizzle the dressing and stir to mix.
- Before serving, top with crumbled feta cheese, if desired.

Salmon Salad with Avocado Dressing

Ingredients:

- Grilled or baked salmon fillet, flaked
- Mixed salad greens
- Cherry tomatoes, halved
- Cucumber, sliced
- Red onion, thinly sliced
- Avocado
- Fresh dill, chopped
- Lemon juice
- Extra virgin olive oil
- Salt and pepper

Steps

- The salad greens, cherry tomatoes, cucumber, and red onion should all be combined in a big salad dish.
- To prepare the dressing, combine the avocado, fresh dill, lemon juice, olive oil, salt, and pepper in a blender or food processor and process until smooth and creamy.

- Toss the salad with the flaked salmon, then top with the avocado dressing.
- Serve after gently tossing to coat.

Eggplant Parmesan

Ingredients:

- Eggplant, sliced into rounds
- All-purpose flour
- Eggs, beaten
- Breadcrumbs
- Grated Parmesan cheese
- Marinara sauce
- Mozzarella cheese, sliced
- Fresh basil leaves
- Olive oil
- Salt and pepper

Steps

- Set the oven's temperature to 375°F (190°C).
- Salt and pepper the slices of eggplant.
- Each slice should be floured, then dipped in beaten eggs before being covered in breadcrumbs and grated Parmesan cheese.
- Over medium-high heat, warm up the olive oil in a big skillet.
- Slices of breaded eggplant should be browned on all sides in a skillet.
- Sliced, cooked eggplant should be placed in a baking dish.
- Each piece is garnished with mozzarella cheese, marinara sauce, and fresh basil.
- Bake for 15 to 20 minutes in the oven, or until the cheese is melted and bubbling.

Asian-inspired Rice Noodle Salad

Ingredients:

- Rice noodles, cooked and drained
- Shredded chicken or tofu
- Shredded carrots
- Red cabbage, thinly sliced
- Bell peppers, thinly sliced
- Fresh cilantro, chopped
- Green onions, sliced
- Lime juice
- Soy sauce or tamari

- Sesame oil
- Honey or maple syrup
- Sesame seeds
- Crushed peanuts (optional)

Steps
- Rice noodles that have been cooked, shredded chicken or tofu, carrots, red cabbage, bell peppers, cilantro, and green onions should all be combined in a big dish.
- To prepare the dressing, combine the lime juice, soy sauce, sesame oil, honey, or maple syrup in a small bowl.
- The dressing should be drizzled over the noodle salad and combined.
- Optional: Before serving, top with crushed peanuts.

Caprese Stuffed Portobello Mushrooms
Ingredients:

- Portobello mushrooms, stems removed
- Fresh mozzarella cheese, sliced
- Cherry tomatoes, halved
- Fresh basil leaves
- Balsamic vinegar
- Olive oil
- Salt and pepper

Steps
- Set the oven's temperature to 400°F (200°C).
- The portobello mushrooms should be put on a baking pan.
- Inside each mushroom, arrange slices of fresh mozzarella cheese, cherry tomato halves, and fresh basil leaves.
- Olive oil and balsamic vinegar should be drizzled over the mushrooms.
- Add salt and pepper to taste.
- Bake for 15 to 20 minutes in the oven, or until the cheese is melted and the mushrooms are cooked through.

Mexican Quinoa Stuffed Bell Peppers
Ingredients:

- Bell peppers, halved and seeds removed
- Cooked quinoa
- Black beans, drained and rinsed

- Corn kernels
- Diced tomatoes
- Red onion, diced
- Ground cumin
- Chili powder
- Paprika
- Salt and pepper
- Shredded cheddar cheese
- Fresh cilantro, chopped

Steps
- Set the oven's temperature to 375°F (190°C).
- Combine the cooked quinoa, black beans, corn, tomatoes, red onion, cumin, chili powder, paprika, salt, and pepper in a sizable bowl.
- The quinoa mixture should be placed inside each bell pepper half.
- The stuffed bell peppers should be put on a baking pan.
- Add some cheddar cheese shavings on top.
- Bake in the oven for 20 to 25 minutes, or until the cheese is melted and bubbling and the peppers are soft.
- Before serving, garnish with fresh cilantro.

Tuna and White Bean Salad

Ingredients:

- Canned tuna, drained
- White beans, rinsed and drained
- Red onion, finely chopped
- Cherry tomatoes, halved
- Kalamata olives
- Fresh parsley, chopped
- Lemon juice
- Extra virgin olive oil
- Salt and pepper

Steps
- The tuna, white beans, red onion, cherry tomatoes, olives, and fresh parsley should all be combined in a big bowl.
- To create the dressing, combine the lemon juice, olive oil, salt, and pepper in a small bowl.
- Over the salad, drizzle the dressing, and mix to blend.

- Offer cold.

Roasted Vegetable Wrap

Ingredients:

- Assorted vegetables (such as bell peppers, zucchini, eggplant, and onions)
- Whole wheat tortilla wraps
- Hummus
- Fresh spinach leaves
- Feta cheese, crumbled
- Fresh herbs (such as basil or parsley)

Steps

- Set the oven's temperature to 400°F (200°C).
- Spread the vegetables out on a baking sheet after tossing them with olive oil, salt, and pepper.
- The veggies should be roasted in the oven for around 20 minutes, or until they are soft and just browned.
- The taco wraps should be warmed.
- Each wrap should have hummus spread on it. Roasted veggies, spinach leaves, feta cheese, and fresh herbs can then be added.
- Enjoy the wraps after carefully rolling them.

Butternut Squash Soup

Ingredients:

- Butternut squash, peeled, seeded, and cubed
- Onion, chopped
- Garlic, minced
- Vegetable broth
- Ground nutmeg
- Ground cinnamon
- Salt and pepper
- Greek yogurt (optional)
- Pumpkin seeds (optional)

Steps

- The onion and garlic should be cooked till tender in a big pot.
- Put the butternut squash in the pot along with the vegetable broth, nutmeg, cinnamon, salt, and pepper.

- Once the mixture has boiled, turn down the heat, cover, and simmer the stew for 20 to 25 minutes, or until the squash is soft.
- To purée the mixture into a smooth, creamy consistency, either use an immersion blender or transfer it to a blender.
- If necessary, adjust the seasoning.
- Optional: Place a dollop of Greek yogurt and some pumpkin seeds on top before serving.

Shrimp Stir-Fry with Vegetables

Ingredients:

- Shrimp, peeled and deveined
- Assorted vegetables (such as bell peppers, broccoli, snap peas, and carrots), sliced or diced
- Garlic, minced
- Ginger, grated
- Soy sauce or tamari
- Sesame oil
- Honey or maple syrup
- Cornstarch
- Cooked brown rice or quinoa

Steps
- To make the sauce, combine the soy sauce, sesame oil, honey or maple syrup, and cornstarch in a small basin.
- In a sizable skillet or wok, heat the oil over medium-high heat.
- Stir-fry the grated ginger and minced garlic in the skillet for one minute, or until fragrant.
- The shrimp should be cooked thoroughly and pink after being added.
- The shrimp should be taken out of the skillet and put aside.
- Then stir-fry the vegetables in the skillet until they are crisp-tender.
- Add the sauce to the skillet with the shrimp and vegetables, then add the shrimp back in.
- Once the sauce has thickened, stir-fry for one more minute.
- Serve with cooked quinoa or brown rice.

Greek Lemon Chicken Skewers

Ingredients:

- Chicken breast, cut into cubes
- Lemon juice
- Garlic, minced
- Fresh oregano, chopped

- Salt and pepper
- Olive oil
- Greek yogurt (for serving, optional)
- Fresh mint leaves (for serving, optional)

Steps

- To make the marinade, combine the lemon juice, minced garlic, oregano, salt, and pepper in a bowl.
- Chicken cubes should be added to the marinade and coated.
- For at least 30 minutes, cover and marinate in the fridge.
- The grill or grill pan should be preheated to medium-high heat.
- Chicken cubes that have been marinated are skewered.
- Until the chicken is thoroughly cooked and slightly browned, grill the skewers for 10 to 12 minutes, flipping once.
- If preferred, garnish with Greek yogurt and fresh mint leaves.

Vegetable Curry

Ingredients:

- Assorted vegetables (such as cauliflower, carrots, peas, and bell peppers), chopped
- Onion, chopped
- Garlic, minced
- Ginger, grated
- Curry powder
- Ground cumin
- Ground coriander
- Turmeric
- Coconut milk
- Vegetable broth
- Salt and pepper
- Fresh cilantro, chopped
- Cooked rice or naan bread

Steps

- Sauté the onion, garlic, and ginger in a big pot until they are tender.
- In the pot, combine the chopped veggies with the curry powder, cumin, coriander, turmeric, salt, and pepper.
- Stirring helps the spices adhere to the vegetables.
- Vegetable broth and coconut milk should be added.

- When the vegetables are cooked, turn down the heat and simmer the mixture for 15 to 20 minutes.
- If necessary, adjust the seasoning.
- With naan bread or cooked rice, serve the vegetable curry.
- Before serving, garnish with fresh cilantro.

Zucchini Noodles with Pesto

Ingredients:

- Zucchini, spiralized into noodles
- Cherry tomatoes, halved
- Pine nuts, toasted
- Fresh basil leaves
- Parmesan cheese, grated
- Garlic, minced
- Lemon juice
- Extra virgin olive oil
- Salt and pepper

Steps
- Olive oil should be heated in a big skillet over a medium heat.
- When aromatic, add the minced garlic and simmer for one minute.
- The spiralized zucchini noodles should be added to the skillet and cooked for two to three minutes, or until just softened.
- Cherry tomato halves, toasted pine nuts, fresh basil leaves, grated Parmesan cheese, lemon juice, salt, and pepper are added after the skillet has been taken off the heat.
- Combine by tossing.
- Serve right away.

Chicken Caesar Salad

Ingredients:

- Grilled or baked chicken breast, sliced
- Romaine lettuce, chopped
- Croutons
- Shredded Parmesan cheese
- Caesar dressing
- Lemon juice
- Salt and pepper

Steps

- Combine the romaine lettuce, croutons, and Parmesan cheese in a sizable salad bowl.
- Sliced grilled chicken breast should be added to the salad.
- Lemon juice and Caesar dressing should be drizzled over the salad.
- To coat, gently toss.
- To taste, add salt and pepper to the food.

Moroccan Chickpea Stew

Ingredients:

- Chickpeas, cooked and drained
- Onion, chopped
- Garlic, minced
- Carrots, diced
- Bell peppers, diced
- Diced tomatoes
- Ground cumin
- Ground coriander
- Ground cinnamon
- Ground turmeric
- Vegetable broth
- Fresh parsley, chopped
- Lemon juice
- Olive oil
- Salt and pepper

Steps

- The chopped onion and minced garlic should be cooked till tender in a big pot.
- Add the ground cumin, coriander, cinnamon, turmeric, salt, and pepper to the saucepan along with the diced carrots, bell peppers, and tomatoes.
- Stirring helps the spices adhere to the vegetables.
- Bring the mixture to a boil after adding the veggie broth.
- Once the vegetables are cooked, lower the heat and let the mixture simmer for around 20 to 25 minutes.
- The cooked chickpeas should be added to the pot and heated well for a further 5 minutes.
- Add lemon juice and fresh parsley after mixing.
- Olive oil should be drizzled before serving.

Shrimp and Avocado Salad

Ingredients:

- Shrimp, peeled and deveined
- Mixed salad greens
- Avocado, sliced
- Cherry tomatoes, halved
- Cucumber, sliced
- Red onion, thinly sliced
- Lemon juice
- Extra virgin olive oil
- Salt and pepper

Steps

- Salt and pepper are used to season the shrimp.
- In a skillet, heat the olive oil over medium-high heat.
- Cook the shrimp in the skillet until they are fully cooked and pink.
- Combine the mixed salad greens, diced avocado, cherry tomatoes, cucumber, and red onion in a large salad bowl.
- To create the dressing, combine the lemon juice, olive oil, salt, and pepper in a small bowl.
- After mixing in the cooked shrimp, cover the salad with the dressing.
- Serve after gently tossing to coat.

Lentil and Vegetable Curry

Ingredients:

- Lentils, cooked
- Assorted vegetables (such as cauliflower, carrots, and peas), chopped
- Onion, chopped
- Garlic, minced
- Ginger, grated
- Curry powder
- Ground cumin
- Ground coriander
- Turmeric
- Coconut milk
- Vegetable broth
- Salt and pepper
- Fresh cilantro, chopped
- Cooked rice or naan bread

Steps

- Sauté the onion, garlic, and ginger in a big pot until they are tender.
- In the pot, combine the chopped veggies with the curry powder, cumin, coriander, turmeric, salt, and pepper.
- Stirring helps the spices adhere to the vegetables.
- Vegetable broth and coconut milk should be added.
- When the vegetables are cooked, turn down the heat and simmer the mixture for 15 to 20 minutes.
- The cooked lentils are then added and heated through by simmering for an additional 5 minutes.
- If necessary, adjust the seasoning.
- Alternatively, serve the lentil and vegetable curry with naan bread and boiled rice.
- Before serving, garnish with fresh cilantro.

Quinoa and Roasted Vegetable Salad

Ingredients:

- Cooked quinoa
- Assorted roasted vegetables (such as sweet potatoes, bell peppers, zucchini, and onions), chopped
- Cherry tomatoes, halved
- Feta cheese, crumbled
- Fresh parsley, chopped
- Lemon juice
- Extra virgin olive oil
- Salt and pepper

Steps

- The cooked quinoa, roasted veggies, cherry tomatoes, feta cheese, and fresh parsley should all be combined in a big bowl.
- To create the dressing, combine the lemon juice, olive oil, salt, and pepper in a small bowl.
- Over the salad, drizzle the dressing, and mix to blend.
- Offer cold.

Turkey and Cranberry Wrap

Ingredients:

- Sliced turkey breast
- Whole wheat tortilla wrap

- Cream cheese
- Cranberry sauce
- Baby spinach leaves
- Sliced almonds

Steps
- Tostada wraps should be evenly spread with cream cheese and cranberry sauce.
- Baby spinach leaves, sliced almonds, and sliced turkey breast are arranged on top.
- Enjoy after securely rolling up the wrap.

Minestrone Soup

Ingredients:

- Vegetable broth
- Onion, chopped
- Garlic, minced
- Carrots, diced
- Celery, diced
- Zucchini, diced
- Canned diced tomatoes
- Kidney beans, rinsed and drained
- Pasta (such as small shells or macaroni)
- Fresh basil leaves, chopped
- Fresh parsley, chopped
- Salt and pepper
- Grated Parmesan cheese (optional)

Steps
- The chopped onion and minced garlic should be cooked till tender in a big pot.
- Add the kidney beans, vegetable broth, salt, and pepper to the saucepan along with the sliced carrots, celery, zucchini, tomatoes, and kidney beans.
- When the vegetables are cooked, turn down the heat and simmer the mixture for 20 to 25 minutes.
- When the pasta is al dente, add it to the pot and cook it as directed on the package.
- Add fresh parsley and basil.
- If necessary, adjust the seasoning.
- Serve with a sprinkle of grated Parmesan cheese, if desired.

Teriyaki Tofu Stir-Fry

Ingredients:

- Extra-firm tofu, cubed
- Assorted vegetables (such as bell peppers, broccoli, snap peas, and carrots), sliced or diced
- Garlic, minced
- Ginger, grated
- Teriyaki sauce
- Soy sauce or tamari
- Sesame oil
- Olive oil
- Cooked brown rice or quinoa

Steps

- To make the marinade, mix the teriyaki sauce, soy sauce, sesame oil, chopped garlic, and grated ginger in a bowl.
- Toss the tofu cubes in the marinade to evenly coat them.
- For at least 30 minutes, cover and marinate in the fridge.
- In a sizable skillet or wok, heat the olive oil over medium-high heat.
- Tofu that has been marinated is added to the skillet and cooked until browned all over.
- Tofu should be taken out of the skillet and placed aside.
- Then stir-fry the vegetables in the skillet until they are crisp-tender.
- Put the tofu back in the skillet with the vegetables and cover with the teriyaki sauce.
- Once the sauce has thickened, stir-fry for one more minute.
- Serve with cooked quinoa or brown rice.

Sweet Potato and Black Bean Burrito

Ingredients:

- Cooked sweet potatoes, mashed
- Black beans, cooked and drained
- Whole wheat tortilla wrap
- Salsa
- Avocado, sliced
- Fresh cilantro, chopped

Steps

- Tostada wrap should be covered in sweet potato mash.
- Include black beans, salsa, avocado slices, and cilantro.
- Enjoy the burrito after a tight roll.

Mediterranean Quinoa Salad

Ingredients:

- Cooked quinoa
- Cucumber, diced
- Cherry tomatoes, halved
- Kalamata olives
- Red onion, thinly sliced
- Fresh parsley, chopped
- Fresh mint leaves, chopped
- Lemon juice
- Extra virgin olive oil
- Salt and pepper
- Crumbled feta cheese (optional)

Steps

- Put the cooked quinoa, sliced cucumber, cherry tomato halves, kalamata olives, red onion slices, fresh parsley, and fresh mint leaves in a sizable bowl.
- To create the dressing, combine the lemon juice, olive oil, salt, and pepper in a small bowl.
- Over the salad, drizzle the dressing, and mix to blend.
- Before serving, top with crumbled feta cheese, if desired.

Tofu and Vegetable Stir-Fry

Ingredients:

- Extra-firm tofu, cubed
- Assorted vegetables (such as bell peppers, broccoli, snap peas, and carrots), sliced or diced
- Garlic, minced
- Ginger, grated
- Soy sauce or tamari
- Sesame oil
- Olive oil
- Cooked brown rice or quinoa

Steps

- Cut the tofu into cubes after pressing it to eliminate more moisture.
- Olive oil should be heated over medium-high heat in a sizable skillet or wok.
- Tofu cubes should be added to the skillet and cooked until evenly browned.
- Tofu should be taken out of the skillet and placed aside.

- The sliced or diced veggies, minced garlic, and grated ginger should all be placed in the same skillet.
- Vegetables should be stir-fried until crisp-tender.
- Put the tofu back in the skillet and cover the tofu and vegetables with soy sauce, tamari, and sesame oil.
- Add another minute of stirring to help the flavors blend.
- Serve with cooked quinoa or brown rice.

Take pleasure in your filling lunch!

Dinner Recipes

Lemon Garlic Salmon:

Ingredients:
- 4 salmon fillets
- 2 tablespoons olive oil
- 2 cloves garlic, minced
- Juice of 1 lemon
- Salt and pepper to taste
- Fresh dill for garnish

steps
- Preheat the oven to 400 degrees Fahrenheit (200 degrees Celsius).
- Combine olive oil, minced garlic, lemon juice, salt, and pepper in a small bowl.
- Line a baking sheet with parchment paper and place the salmon fillets on it.
- Brush the garlic-lemon mixture over the fish.
- Bake for 12-15 minutes, or until the salmon is well cooked.
- Serve garnished with fresh dill.

Balsamic Chicken with Roasted Vegetables:

Ingredients:

- 4 chicken breasts
- 1/4 cup balsamic vinegar
- 2 tablespoons olive oil
- 2 tablespoons honey

- 1 teaspoon dried thyme
- Salt and pepper to taste
- Assorted vegetables (such as bell peppers, zucchini, and cherry tomatoes)

steps

- Preheat the oven to 400 degrees Fahrenheit (200 degrees Celsius).
- Whisk together the balsamic vinegar, olive oil, honey, dried thyme, salt, and pepper in a small bowl.
- Place the chicken breasts in a baking dish and evenly coat with the balsamic mixture.
- Arrange the vegetables in a circle around the chicken.
- Bake for 25-30 minutes, or until the chicken is thoroughly cooked and the vegetables are soft.
- Serve the chicken with vegetables that have been cooked.

Quinoa Stuffed Bell Peppers:

Ingredients:

- 4 bell peppers
- 1 cup cooked quinoa
- 1 cup black beans, rinsed and drained
- 1 cup diced tomatoes
- 1/2 cup corn kernels
- 1/4 cup chopped fresh cilantro
- 1 teaspoon cumin
- 1/2 teaspoon paprika
- Salt and pepper to taste
- Shredded cheese (optional)

steps

- Preheat the oven to 350°F/175°C.
- Remove the tops of the bell peppers and the seeds and membranes.
- Combine cooked quinoa, black beans, chopped tomatoes, corn kernels, cilantro, cumin, paprika, salt, and pepper in a mixing dish.
- Fill the bell peppers to the brim with the quinoa mixture.
- Cover the filled bell peppers in a baking dish with foil.
- Bake for 30 minutes, then remove the foil and continue baking for another 10 minutes.
- If preferred, top the peppers with shredded cheese and bake for another 5 minutes, or until the cheese is melted and bubbling.

Serve the quinoa-stuffed bell peppers immediately.

Teriyaki Stir-Fry with Tofu and Vegetables:

Ingredients:

- 14 oz (400g) extra firm tofu, drained and cubed
- 2 tablespoons soy sauce
- 2 tablespoons teriyaki sauce
- 1 tablespoon sesame oil
- 1 tablespoon cornstarch
- 1 tablespoon vegetable oil
- 2 cloves garlic, minced
- 1 tablespoon grated ginger
- Assorted vegetables (such as broccoli, bell peppers, and carrots)
- Cooked rice or noodles for serving

Steps
- Add the soy sauce, teriyaki sauce, sesame oil, and cornstarch in a mixing bowl. Combine thoroughly.
- In a large skillet or wok, heat the vegetable oil over medium heat.
- Cook for 1 minute, or until the minced garlic and grated ginger are aromatic.
- Cook until the tofu cubes are lightly browned on both sides in the skillet.
- Stir-fry the veggies for 4-5 minutes, or until crisp-tender.
- Toss the tofu and veggies with the teriyaki sauce mixture.
- Cook for a further 2-3 minutes, or until the sauce thickens, stirring constantly.
- Over cooked rice or noodles, serve the teriyaki stir-fry.

Mediterranean Chickpea Salad:

Ingredients:

- 2 cups cooked chickpeas (or canned, rinsed and drained)
- 1 cup cherry tomatoes, halved
- 1 cucumber, diced
- 1/2 red onion, thinly sliced
- 1/4 cup Kalamata olives, pitted and halved
- 1/4 cup crumbled feta cheese
- 2 tablespoons extra virgin olive oil
- 1 tablespoon lemon juice
- 1 teaspoon dried oregano
- Salt and pepper to taste

steps

- Combine the chickpeas, Kalamata olives, cucumber, red onion, cherry tomatoes, and crumbled feta cheese in a big bowl.
-
- Whisk together the extra virgin olive oil, lemon juice, dried oregano, salt, and pepper in a separate small bowl.
- Toss the chickpea salad carefully with the dressing to coat.
- Allow the salad to marinate for at least 30 minutes in the refrigerator to allow the flavors to mingle.
- As a light and nutritious supper alternative, serve the Mediterranean chickpea salad.

Grilled Lemon Herb Chicken:

Ingredients:

- 4 boneless, skinless chicken breasts
- 2 lemons, juiced and zested
- 2 tablespoons olive oil
- 2 cloves garlic, minced
- 1 tablespoon chopped fresh thyme
- 1 tablespoon chopped fresh rosemary
- Salt and pepper to taste

step
- Set the grill's temperature to medium-high.
- Combine the lemon juice, lemon zest, olive oil, minced garlic, chopped thyme, chopped rosemary, salt, and pepper in a small mixing bowl.
- Put the chicken breasts in a shallow dish, and then cover them with the lemon-herb marinade.
- Give the chicken at least 30 minutes to marinate.
- The chicken breasts should be cooked through and the juices flow clear after grilling for 6 to 8 minutes on each side.
- Before serving, take the chicken from the grill and allow it to rest for a while.
- Your choice of side dishes should go with the grilled lemon herb chicken.

Lentil Curry with Coconut Milk:

Ingredients:

- 1 cup dried red lentils
- 1 onion, finely chopped

- 2 cloves garlic, minced
- 1 tablespoon grated ginger
- 1 tablespoon curry powder
- 1 teaspoon ground cumin
- 1 teaspoon ground turmeric
- 1 can (14 oz/400ml) coconut milk
- 1 can (14 oz/400g) diced tomatoes
- 1 cup vegetable broth
- 1 tablespoon olive oil
- Fresh cilantro for garnish
- Cooked rice or naan bread for serving

steps

- Lentils should be rinsed in cold water and laid aside.
- In a big saucepan, warm up the olive oil over medium heat.
- Add the minced garlic, grated ginger, and the diced onion. Sauté until aromatic for two to three minutes.
- Turmeric, cumin, and curry powder should all be added to the saucepan. As you stir, sprinkle the spices over the onion mixture.
- In the saucepan, combine the lentils, coconut milk, chopped tomatoes, and vegetable broth.
- When the lentils are soft and the flavors are blended, bring the stew to a boil, then lower the heat to a simmer for 20 to 25 minutes.
- Serve the hot lentil stew with naan bread or over hot rice. Add fresh cilantro as a garnish.

Shrimp Scampi Pasta:

Ingredients:

- 8 oz (225g) spaghetti or linguine pasta
- 1 lb (450g) shrimp, peeled and deveined
- 4 cloves garlic, minced
- 2 tablespoons lemon juice
- 1/4 cup white wine (optional)
- 2 tablespoons unsalted butter
- 2 tablespoons olive oil
- 1/4 teaspoon red pepper flakes (optional)
- Salt and pepper to taste
- Chopped parsley for garnish

steps

- Pasta should be cooked as directed on the package until it is al dente. Drain, then set apart.
- Melt butter and extra virgin olive oil in a big pan over medium heat.
- Red pepper flakes (if used) and minced garlic are added to the skillet. Sauté until fragrant for one minute.
- When the shrimp are pink and cooked through, add them to the skillet and cook for two to three minutes on each side.
- Add the white wine and lemon juice, if desired. To enable the flavors to combine, cook for one more minute.
- To taste, add salt and pepper to the food.
- Toss the cooked pasta with the sauce and shrimp in the skillet after adding it.
- Serve the shrimp scampi pasta right away after adding some chopped parsley as a garnish.

Spinach and Feta Stuffed Chicken Breast:

Ingredients:

- 4 boneless, skinless chicken breasts
- 1 cup fresh spinach leaves
- 1/2 cup crumbled feta cheese
- 2 cloves garlic, minced
- 1 tablespoon olive oil
- Salt and pepper to taste

Steps:

- Set the oven's temperature to 400°F (200°C).
- Cut horizontally through the side of each chicken breast, taking careful not to cut all the way through.
- Olive oil is heated in a pan at a medium temperature.
- Sauté the minced garlic for 1 minute, or until aromatic.
- Cook until wilted after adding fresh spinach leaves to the pan.
- Turn off the heat and let the spinach gradually cool.
- The feta cheese crumbles and wilted spinach should be combined in a dish.
- Place the spinach and feta mixture into each chicken breast, and if necessary, fasten with toothpicks.
- Salt and pepper the chicken breasts that have been stuffed.
- An oven-safe nonstick skillet is warmed over medium-high heat.
- The filled chicken breasts should be browned for 2-3 minutes on each side.

- When the chicken is cooked through and the juices run clear, place the pan in the preheated oven and bake for 15-20 minutes.
- Before serving the chicken breast packed with spinach and feta, take out the toothpicks, if any.

Beef Stir-Fry with Broccoli and Mushrooms:

Ingredients:

- 1 lb (450g) beef sirloin, thinly sliced
- 2 cups broccoli florets
- 1 cup sliced mushrooms
- 1 onion, sliced
- 2 cloves garlic, minced
- 2 tablespoons soy sauce
- 1 tablespoon oyster sauce
- 1 tablespoon cornstarch
- 1 tablespoon vegetable oil
- Salt and pepper to taste
- Cooked rice or noodles for serving

Steps:

- Mix the soy sauce, oyster sauce, cornstarch, salt, and pepper in a small basin. Place aside.
- In a large skillet or wok, heat vegetable oil over high heat.
- To the skillet, add sliced onion and minced garlic. Stir-fry the onions for one to two minutes, or until aromatic.
- Sweat the beef slices in the pan for two to three minutes, or until browned.
- Sliced mushrooms and broccoli florets should be added to the skillet. Vegetables should be stir-fried for 3–4 minutes to get a crisp–tender state.
- Over the meat and veggies, pour the soy sauce mixture.
- Stir-fry the ingredients for a further 2 to 3 minutes, or until the sauce thickens and covers everything.
- Over hot cooked rice or noodles, serve the beef stir-fry.

Baked Eggplant Parmesan:

Ingredients:

- 2 large eggplants, sliced into 1/2-inch rounds

- 2 cups marinara sauce
- 2 cups shredded mozzarella cheese
- 1 cup grated Parmesan cheese
- 1/2 cup breadcrumbs
- 2 tablespoons chopped fresh basil
- 2 tablespoons chopped fresh parsley
- 2 tablespoons olive oil
- Salt and pepper to taste

Steps:

- Set the oven's temperature to 375°F (190°C).
- The eggplant slices should be put on a baking pan with parchment paper.
- Olive oil should be brushed on each slice before being salt and peppered.
- The eggplant slices should be soft and gently brown after 20 to 25 minutes in the oven.
- Spread a thin layer of marinara sauce in a baking dish.
- Slices of cooked eggplant should be arranged in a single layer on top of the sauce.
- Over the eggplant, scatter a layer of breadcrumbs, mozzarella cheese, grated Parmesan cheese, chopped basil, and chopped parsley.
- Up until all the components have been utilized, repeat the layering process, capping it off with a sauce and cheese layer.
- Bake for 20 minutes with the foil covering the baking dish.
- In order to get the cheese to melt and bubble, bake for an extra 10 minutes after removing the foil.
- Before serving, let the baked eggplant Parmesan cool for a while.

Thai Red Curry with Vegetables and Tofu:

Ingredients:

- 14 oz (400g) firm tofu, cubed
- 2 cups mixed vegetables (such as bell peppers, snow peas, and carrots)
- 1 can (14 oz/400ml) coconut milk
- 2 tablespoons Thai red curry paste
- 1 tablespoon soy sauce
- 1 tablespoon brown sugar
- 1 tablespoon vegetable oil
- Fresh cilantro for garnish
- Cooked rice for serving

Steps:

- Over medium heat, warm vegetable oil in a large skillet or wok.
- Cubed tofu should be added to the skillet and cooked until just faintly browned all over. Take out of the skillet, then set it aside.
- Add the mixed veggies to the same pan and stir-fry for 3–4 minutes, or until crisp–tender.
- Mix the coconut milk, soy sauce, brown sugar, and Thai red curry paste in a small bowl.
- Fill the pan with the veggies and the coconut milk mixture.
- Stir everything together before adding the tofu back to the skillet.
- The curry mixture should be cooked through and the flavors blended after 5-7 minutes of simmering.
- Thai red curry should be served over cooked rice and should be garnished with fresh cilantro.

Moroccan Spiced Roasted Vegetables:

Ingredients:

- 2 cups mixed vegetables (such as carrots, zucchini, bell peppers, and onions), cut into bite-sized pieces
- 2 tablespoons olive oil
- 1 tablespoon honey
- 1 teaspoon ground cumin
- 1 teaspoon ground coriander
- 1/2 teaspoon ground cinnamon
- 1/4 teaspoon ground paprika
- Salt and pepper to taste
- Fresh parsley for garnish

Steps:

- Set the oven's temperature to 425°F (220°C).
- Mix the olive oil, honey, cinnamon, ground paprika, ground cumin, ground coriander, ground paprika, salt, and pepper in a large bowl.
- Toss the dish of mixed veggies with the spice mixture to evenly coat them.
- On a baking sheet covered with parchment paper, arrange the veggies in a single layer.
- When the veggies are soft and just beginning to caramelize, roast them in the preheated oven for 25 to 30 minutes, stirring once halfway through.
- Before serving, take the dish out of the oven and top with fresh parsley.

Stuffed Bell Peppers with Ground Turkey and Quinoa:

Ingredients:

- 4 bell peppers
- 1 lb (450g) ground turkey
- 1 cup cooked quinoa
- 1 onion, finely chopped
- 2 cloves garlic, minced
- 1 can (14 oz/400g) diced tomatoes
- 1 teaspoon dried oregano
- 1/2 teaspoon dried basil
- 1/4 teaspoon red pepper flakes (optional)
- Salt and pepper to taste
- Shredded cheese for topping (optional)

Steps:
- Set the oven's temperature to 375°F (190°C).
- Remove the bell peppers' tops, then scoop out the seeds and membranes.
- The ground turkey should be cooked until browned and no longer pink in a large pan over medium heat. Remove any extra fat.
- To the pan containing the ground turkey, add the minced garlic and chopped onion. The onion should be transparent after 2 to 3 minutes of sautéing.
- Cooked quinoa, diced tomatoes (with juice), dried oregano, dry basil, red pepper flakes (if used), salt, and pepper are all added in a final stirring. Stirring often, cook for a further 2 to 3 minutes.
- Pack the ground turkey and quinoa mixture snugly within the bell peppers.
- The filled bell peppers should be put on a baking dish. Shredded cheese can be added to the peppers' tops if preferred.
- Bake the bell peppers for 25 to 30 minutes, or until they are soft and the filling is well cooked.
- Before serving, let the filled bell peppers cool for a while.

Honey Mustard Glazed Salmon:

Ingredients:

- 4 salmon fillets
- 3 tablespoons Dijon mustard
- 2 tablespoons honey
- 1 tablespoon olive oil
- 1 tablespoon fresh lemon juice
- Salt and pepper to taste

Steps:

- Set the oven's temperature to 400°F (200°C).
- Mix Dijon mustard, honey, olive oil, lemon juice, salt, and pepper in a small bowl.
- Salmon fillets should be put on a baking pan covered with parchment paper.
- Apply a uniform layer of honey mustard glaze on the fish.
- When the salmon is cooked through and flakes readily with a fork, bake for 12 to 15 minutes.
- Your choice of side dishes should go with the salmon with the honey mustard glaze.

Chicken and Vegetable Stir-Fry:

Ingredients:

- 4 boneless, skinless chicken breasts, cut into strips
- 2 cups mixed vegetables (such as bell peppers, broccoli, carrots, and snap peas)
- 3 tablespoons soy sauce
- 2 tablespoons oyster sauce
- 1 tablespoon cornstarch
- 1 tablespoon vegetable oil
- 2 cloves garlic, minced
- Salt and pepper to taste
- Cooked rice or noodles for serving

Steps:

- In a small mixing bowl, combine soy sauce, oyster sauce, cornstarch, salt, and pepper. Place aside.
- In a large skillet or wok, heat vegetable oil over high heat.
- Stir in the minced garlic and cook for one minute, or until fragrant.
- Cook the chicken strips in the skillet until well-browned and done.
- When the mixed veggies are crisp-tender, add them to the pan and stir-fry for 3–4 minutes.
- Over the chicken and veggies, pour the soy sauce concoction.
- Stir-fry the ingredients for a further 2 to 3 minutes, or until the sauce thickens and covers everything.
- Over hot cooked rice or noodles, serve the stir-fried chicken and vegetables.

Baked Ziti:

Ingredients:

- 8 oz (225g) ziti pasta
- 1 lb (450g) ground beef or Italian sausage
- 1 onion, chopped

- 2 cloves garlic, minced
- 2 cups marinara sauce
- 1 cup shredded mozzarella cheese
- 1/2 cup grated Parmesan cheese
- 1 tablespoon olive oil
- 1 teaspoon dried oregano
- 1/2 teaspoon dried basil
- Salt and pepper to taste

Steps:

- Set the oven's temperature to 375°F (190°C).
- Ziti pasta should be prepared as directed on the package until it is al dente. Drain, then set apart.
- Olive oil should be heated in a large pan over a medium heat.
- Add minced garlic and sliced onion to the skillet. For 2-3 minutes, sauté until aromatic and the onions are just beginning to soften.
- Cook until browned by adding ground beef or Italian sausage to the skillet. Remove any extra fat.
- Add salt, pepper, dried basil, dry oregano, and marinara sauce. For the flavors to combine, simmer for 5 minutes.
- Spread a thin layer of the beef sauce in a big baking dish.
- Ziti pasta that has been cooked should be layered over the sauce.
- Over the noodles, smear a layer of grated Parmesan cheese and mozzarella cheese.
- Up until all the components have been utilized, repeat the layering process, capping it off with a sauce and cheese layer.
- Bake for 20 minutes with the foil covering the baking dish.
- In order to get the cheese to melt and bubble, bake for an extra 10 minutes after removing the foil.
- Prior to serving, let the baked ziti cool for a few minutes..

Teriyaki Salmon with Steamed Vegetables:

Ingredients:

- 4 salmon fillets
- 1/4 cup soy sauce
- 2 tablespoons honey
- 1 tablespoon rice vinegar
- 1 tablespoon sesame oil
- 2 cloves garlic, minced
- 1 teaspoon grated ginger
- 2 cups mixed vegetables (such as broccoli, carrots, and snap peas)

- Salt and pepper to taste

Steps:

- Set the oven's temperature to 400°F (200°C).
- Soy sauce, honey, rice vinegar, sesame oil, chopped garlic, and grated ginger should all be combined in a small bowl.
- Put the salmon fillets in a baking dish, then equally distribute the teriyaki sauce mixture over them. For 15 minutes, marinate.
- For 12 to 15 minutes, or until the salmon is cooked through and flakes readily with a fork, bake the salmon in the preheated oven.
- Steam the mixed veggies until crisp-tender while the salmon bakes.
- Add salt and pepper to the cooked veggies.
-
- Steamed veggies should be served alongside the salmon teriyaki.

Mushroom and Spinach Risotto:

Ingredients:

- 1 cup Arborio rice
- 4 cups vegetable broth
- 1 onion, chopped
- 2 cloves garlic, minced
- 8 oz (225g) mushrooms, sliced
- 2 cups fresh spinach leaves
- 1/2 cup grated Parmesan cheese
- 2 tablespoons butter
- 2 tablespoons olive oil
- Salt and pepper to taste

Steps:

- Warm up the veggie broth in a medium saucepan over low heat.
- Melt butter and olive oil in a large pan over medium heat.
- Add minced garlic and sliced onion to the skillet. For 2-3 minutes, sauté until aromatic and onions are just beginning to soften.
- Sliced mushrooms should be added to the skillet and cooked until they give off moisture and become soft.
-
- To evenly coat the rice with the mushroom mixture, toss in the Arborio rice and simmer for a further 1-2 minutes.
- Warm vegetable broth should be added to the skillet approximately 1/2 cup at a time, stirring frequently until the liquid is completely absorbed. Continue doing this for 20 to 25 minutes, or until the rice is creamy and al dente.

- Fresh spinach leaves are added and cooked for a further two to three minutes, or until wilted.
- Add the grated Parmesan cheese after turning off the heat in the skillet.
- To taste, add salt and pepper to the food.
- Prior to serving, let the risotto with mushrooms and spinach have some time to rest.

Baked Chicken Parmesan:
Ingredients:

- 4 boneless, skinless chicken breasts
- 1 cup breadcrumbs
- 1/2 cup grated Parmesan cheese
- 1/2 cup all-purpose flour
- 2 eggs, beaten
- 1 cup marinara sauce
- 1 cup shredded mozzarella cheese
- 2 tablespoons olive oil
- 1 tablespoon chopped fresh basil
- 1 tablespoon chopped fresh parsley
- Salt and pepper to taste

Steps:

- Set the oven's temperature to 375°F (190°C).
- Combine breadcrumbs, Parmesan cheese that has been shredded, salt, and pepper in a shallow dish.
- Place beaten eggs in a third shallow dish, followed by flour.
- Shake off any excess flour after coating each chicken breast.
- The floured chicken breast is then dipped into the beaten eggs, then coated with the breadcrumb mixture and pressed to adhere.
- A big skillet with medium heat is used to heat the olive oil.
- In a pan, add the breaded chicken breasts and cook for two to three minutes on each side, or until golden brown.
- Place the chicken breasts that have been browned in a baking dish.
- Chicken breasts should be covered in marinara sauce and topped with shredded mozzarella cheese.
- Bake for 20 to 25 minutes, or until the cheese is melted and bubbling and the chicken is thoroughly cooked.
- Before serving the baked chicken Parmesan, garnish with fresh basil and parsley.

Shrimp Scampi with Linguine:

Ingredients:

- 1 lb (450g) linguine pasta
- 1 lb (450g) shrimp, peeled and deveined
- 4 cloves garlic, minced
- 1/4 cup butter
- 1/4 cup white wine
- 2 tablespoons lemon juice
- 2 tablespoons chopped fresh parsley
- Salt and pepper to taste
- Red pepper flakes (optional)

Steps:

- As directed on the package, prepare the linguine pasta until it is al dente. Drain, then set apart.
- Melt the butter in a large pan over medium heat.
- Stir in the minced garlic and cook for one minute, or until fragrant.
- When the shrimp are pink and cooked through, add them to the pan and cook for 2–3 minutes.
- White wine and lemon juice should be added and mixed together.
- Add salt, pepper, and red pepper flakes (if using) for seasoning.
-
- Cook for a further 2 to 3 minutes, or until the sauce starts to slightly thicken.
- Toss the shrimp scampi sauce with the cooked linguine.
- Before serving, add some chopped parsley as a garnish.

Teriyaki Vegetable Stir-Fry:

Ingredients:

- 2 cups mixed vegetables (such as broccoli, bell peppers, snap peas, and carrots)
- 1/4 cup soy sauce
- 2 tablespoons honey
- 1 tablespoon rice vinegar
- 1 tablespoon sesame oil
- 2 cloves garlic, minced
- 1 teaspoon grated ginger
- 2 tablespoons vegetable oil
- Cooked rice for serving

Steps:

- In a small bowl, whisk together soy sauce, honey, rice vinegar, sesame oil, minced garlic, and grated ginger. Set aside.
- Heat vegetable oil in a large skillet or wok over high heat.
-
- Add the mixed vegetables to the skillet and stir-fry for 3-4 minutes until crisp-tender.
- Pour the teriyaki sauce mixture over the vegetables and stir to coat.
- Continue to stir-fry for another 2-3 minutes until the sauce thickens and coats the vegetables.
- Serve the teriyaki vegetable stir-fry hot over cooked rice.

Lemon Herb Roasted Chicken:

Ingredients:

- 1 whole chicken, approximately 4 lbs (1.8kg)
- 1 lemon, sliced
- 4 sprigs fresh rosemary
- 4 sprigs fresh thyme
- 4 cloves garlic, minced
- 2 tablespoons olive oil
- Salt and pepper to taste

Steps:
- Set the oven's temperature to 425°F (220°C).
- Chicken should be rinsed and dried with paper towels.
- Add salt, pepper, and minced garlic to the chicken's inside and outside for seasoning.
- Put the lemon slices, fresh thyme, and rosemary within the cavity of the chicken.
-
- Use kitchen thread to bind the legs together.
- Olive oil should be drizzled over the chicken before placing it in a roasting pan.
- The chicken should be roasted in the preheated oven for 1 hour and 15 minutes, or until the juices flow clear and the internal temperature reaches 165°F (74°C).
- After removing the chicken from the oven, give it a 10-minute rest before carving.

Vegetable Curry with Coconut Milk:

Ingredients:

- 2 cups mixed vegetables (such as cauliflower, potatoes, carrots, and peas)
- 1 can (14 oz/400ml) coconut milk
- 1 onion, chopped
- 2 cloves garlic, minced

- 1 tablespoon curry powder
- 1 teaspoon ground cumin
- 1 teaspoon ground coriander
- 1/2 teaspoon turmeric
- 1/4 teaspoon cayenne pepper (optional)
- 2 tablespoons vegetable oil
- Salt and pepper to taste
- Cooked rice or naan bread for serving

Steps:
- Over medium heat, warm vegetable oil in a big saucepan or skillet.
- Add minced garlic and sliced onion to the skillet. For 2-3 minutes, sauté until aromatic and onions are just beginning to soften.
- Add the cayenne pepper (if using), turmeric, curry powder, ground cumin, ground coriander, and so on. The spices should cook for one minute to toast.
- The mixture of veggies should be added to the skillet and cooked for 5 minutes, or until they begin to soften.
- Salt and pepper to taste, add the coconut milk, and then simmer.
- When the veggies are cooked through and the flavors are blended, turn the heat down to low, cover the skillet, and let the curry simmer for 15 to 20 minutes.
- Serve the hot vegetable curry with naan bread or over hot rice.

Baked Stuffed Peppers with Quinoa and Black Beans:

Ingredients:

- 4 bell peppers
- 1 cup cooked quinoa
- 1 can (15 oz/425g) black beans, drained and rinsed
- 1 cup diced tomatoes
- 1/2 cup shredded cheddar cheese
- 1/4 cup chopped fresh cilantro
- 1 tablespoon olive oil
- 1 teaspoon ground cumin
- 1/2 teaspoon chili powder
- Salt and pepper to taste

Steps:
- The oven should be preheated at 375°F (190°C).
- Scoop off the seeds and membranes from the bell peppers after removing the tops.
- In a large dish, add cooked quinoa, black beans, diced tomatoes, cheddar cheese, chopped cilantro, olive oil, cumin powder, chili powder, salt, and pepper. Completely combine.

- In the bell peppers, cram the quinoa and black bean mixture tightly.
- The packed bell peppers should be placed in a baking dish and covered with foil.
- Bake for 25 minutes. Remove the cover and continue baking for a further 10 to 15 minutes, or until the mixture has well heated through and the peppers are tender.
- Allow the stuffed peppers to cool for a time before serving.

Spaghetti Carbonara:

Ingredients:

- 8 oz (225g) spaghetti
- 4 slices bacon, chopped
- 3 cloves garlic, minced
- 2 large eggs
- 1/2 cup grated Parmesan cheese
- 2 tablespoons chopped fresh parsley
- Salt and pepper to taste

Steps:

- As directed on the package, prepare the spaghetti noodle until it is al dente. Drain, then set apart.
- Cook the diced bacon to crispiness over medium heat in a big pan. From the skillet, take out the bacon, and set it aside.
- Sauté the minced garlic in the bacon oil for one minute, or until fragrant, in the same skillet.
- Mix the eggs, Parmesan cheese, salt, and pepper in a medium bowl.
- Cooked spaghetti should be added to the skillet with the garlic and mixed around to evenly distribute the bacon fat.
- While swiftly pouring the egg mixture over the spaghetti and swirling continually until the eggs thicken but do not scramble, remove the pan from the heat.
- Toss the chopped fresh parsley and crispy bacon together in the skillet.

- Serve the spaghetti carbonara right away, topped with more parsley and Parmesan cheese that has been grated.

Baked Salmon with Lemon and Dill:

Ingredients:

- 4 salmon fillets
- 2 lemons, sliced
- 4 sprigs fresh dill

- 2 tablespoons olive oil
- Salt and pepper to taste

Steps:

- Set the oven's temperature to 400°F (200°C).
- Salmon fillets should be put on a baking pan covered with parchment paper.
- Olive oil and salt and pepper should be drizzled over the salmon fillets.
- Each salmon fillet should be topped with lemon slices and fresh dill sprigs.
- To construct a package with the salmon inside, fold the parchment paper's sides over and firmly press them together.
- When the salmon is cooked through and flakes easily with a fork, bake it in the preheated oven for 12 to 15 minutes.
- Before serving, take the salmon packets out of the oven and give them some time to rest.

Thai Green Curry with Chicken:

Ingredients:

- 1 lb (450g) boneless, skinless chicken breasts, cut into bite-sized pieces
- 1 can (14 oz/400ml) coconut milk
- 2 tablespoons Thai green curry paste
- 1 red bell pepper, sliced
- 1 zucchini, sliced
- 1 cup sliced mushrooms
- 1 cup baby corn
- 1 tablespoon fish sauce
- 1 tablespoon lime juice
- 1 tablespoon brown sugar
- 2 tablespoons vegetable oil
- Fresh basil leaves for garnish
- Cooked rice for serving

Steps:

- Over medium heat, warm vegetable oil in a big saucepan or skillet.
- Cook the chicken pieces in the skillet until well-browned and done. The chicken should be taken out of the pan and put aside.
- Thai green curry paste should be added to the same skillet and cooked for one minute to bring out its spices.
- Pour the coconut milk over the curry paste, then whisk.
- Red bell pepper, zucchini, mushrooms, and baby corn should all be added to the skillet. Cook the veggies for 5-7 minutes, or until they are soft.

- Add lime juice, brown sugar, and fish sauce after stirring.
- Re-add the cooked chicken to the skillet and heat through over low heat for an additional two to three minutes.
- Over cooked rice, top the Thai green curry with fresh basil leaves.

Beef Stir-Fry with Broccoli and Ginger:

Ingredients:

- 1 lb (450g) beef sirloin, thinly sliced
- 2 cups broccoli florets
- 1 onion, sliced
- 2 cloves garlic, minced
- 1 tablespoon grated fresh ginger
- 2 tablespoons soy sauce
- 1 tablespoon oyster sauce
- 1 tablespoon cornstarch
- 1 tablespoon vegetable oil
- Salt and pepper to taste
- Cooked rice or noodles for serving

Steps:
- Mix the soy sauce, oyster sauce, cornstarch, salt, and pepper in a small basin. Place aside.
- In a large skillet or wok, heat vegetable oil over high heat.
- Add grated ginger and chopped garlic to the skillet. Sauté until fragrant for one minute.
- Sliced beef should be added to the skillet and cooked throughly.
- Broccoli florets and thinly sliced onion should be added to the skillet and stir-fried for 3 to 4 minutes, or until the veggies are crisp-tender.
- Over the meat and veggies, pour the soy sauce mixture.
- Stir-fry the ingredients for a further 2 to 3 minutes, or until the sauce thickens and covers everything.
- Over hot cooked rice or noodles, serve the beef stir-fry.

Vegetarian Stuffed Bell Peppers:

Ingredients:

- 4 bell peppers
- 1 cup cooked quinoa
- 1 cup black beans, drained and rinsed

- 1 cup corn kernels
- 1/2 cup diced tomatoes
- 1/2 cup shredded Monterey Jack cheese
- 2 tablespoons chopped fresh cilantro
- 1 tablespoon olive oil
- 1 teaspoon ground cumin
- 1/2 teaspoon chili powder
- Salt and pepper to taste

Steps:
- Set the oven's temperature to 375°F (190°C).
- Remove the bell peppers' tops, then scoop out the seeds and membranes.
- Cooked quinoa, black beans, corn, diced tomatoes, shredded Monterey Jack cheese, chopped cilantro, olive oil, cumin, chili powder, salt, and pepper should all be combined in a big dish. Mix thoroughly.
- Pack the quinoa and veggie mixture tightly into the bell peppers.
- In a baking dish, put the filled bell peppers, and cover with foil.
- For 25 minutes, bake. After that, take off the foil and bake for an additional 10 to 15 minutes, or until the mixture is well cooked and the peppers are soft.
- Before serving, let the stuffed peppers cool for a while.

Chapter 6

Wholesome Snacks and Appetizers

Our everyday eating habits include snacking, which gives us an energy boost and satisfies our appetite in between meals. However, it's important to select snacks that enhance our general health and wellbeing in addition to satisfying our desires. Healthy nibbles and starters are a great way to fuel our bodies while savoring mouthwatering tastes and textures.

The emphasis is on using nutrient-dense products that give necessary vitamins, minerals, and antioxidants in healthy snacks and appetizers. These foods are made to feed our bodies, boost our immune systems, and help us control inflammation. This is crucial for seniors since they may be more vulnerable to age-related health concerns.

Prioritizing whole foods and reducing the use of processed and refined components is one of the guiding principles of healthy snacking. Your snack plate should have fresh fruits and vegetables, which offer a variety of vitamins, fiber, and antioxidants. Crunchy carrot sticks, celery with nut butter, or colorful bell pepper slices may all fulfill your want for a pleasing crunch while giving your body essential nutrients.

Another crucial ingredient in healthy snacks and appetizers are nuts and seeds. They satisfy hunger and are a great source of fiber, protein, and healthy fats, as well as a variety of minerals and omega-3 fatty acids. Almonds, walnuts, pumpkin seeds, and sunflower seeds are delicious as standalone snacks or may be added for variety and flavor to homemade trail mixes.

Protein-rich choices like Greek yogurt and cottage cheese may be made into delectable and wholesome snacks. They are delicious on their own, but you can also add fresh berries, granola, or honey to them for sweetness. These dairy products satisfy appetites and offer calcium, probiotics for intestinal health, and a creamy mouthfeel.

Hummus and guacamole are great plant-based options for individuals who are seeking them. Chickpeas are used to make hummus, which is a creamy and tasty dip for whole-grain crackers or veggie sticks that also provides protein and fiber. Avocados are full of vitamins, minerals, and good fats, which are all present in guacamole. It may be spread over toast or sandwiches, or it can be savored with whole-grain tortilla chips.

Granola bars and homemade energy balls are excellent portable snacks. Oats, nuts, seeds, dried fruits, and natural sweeteners like honey or dates can all be used to make them. These homemade sweets deliver prolonged energy and satiate cravings without the use of processed foods or added sugars since they include a balanced blend of carbs, good fats, and protein.

Due to their crisp texture and nutritional content, vegetable-based snacks such as roasted chickpeas or kale chips are becoming more and more popular. Traditional snacks may be replaced with protein-rich roasted chickpeas, while kale chips offer a tasty and healthy way to eat leafy greens. With the ability to be customized with various herbs and spices, these handmade choices let you cater them to your personal tastes.

It's vital to remember that healthy snacking heavily relies on portion management. Despite the fact that these snacks are healthy, ingesting too many of them might result in calorie overload. A balanced diet may be maintained and overindulgence avoided by paying attention to portion sizes and practicing mindful eating.

Finally, healthy snacks and appetizers provide us a chance to fuel our bodies with nutrient-dense products while savoring mouthwatering flavors. We can provide our bodies with the nutrients they need to function properly, support our general health, and maintain an active and vibrant lifestyle by incorporating fresh fruits and vegetables, nuts and seeds, yogurt or cottage cheese, hummus or guacamole, homemade energy balls or granola bars, and vegetable-based snacks into our snacking routine. Snacking may be made enjoyable and nutritious for seniors and people of all ages by embracing these healthy snack alternatives, which can enhance feelings of pleasure and wellbeing.

Recipes

Crunchy Vegetable Sticks with Yogurt Dip:

Ingredients:

- Carrot sticks
- Celery sticks
- Cucumber sticks
- Cherry tomatoes
- Greek yogurt
- Fresh dill
- Lemon juice
- Salt and pepper to taste

steps

- Vegetables should be washed and sliced into sticks.
- Greek yogurt, freshly chopped dill, lemon juice, salt, and pepper should all be combined in a small bowl.
- Serve the yogurt dip alongside the veggie sticks.

Energy Balls:

Ingredients:

- 1 cup oats
- 1/2 cup nut butter (such as almond butter or peanut butter)
- 1/4 cup honey or maple syrup
- 1/4 cup ground flaxseed
- 1/4 cup dark chocolate chips
- 1/4 cup dried fruits (such as raisins or cranberries)
- 1 teaspoon vanilla extract

steps

- Oats, nut butter, honey, maple syrup, ground flaxseed, chocolate chips, dried fruits, and vanilla extract should all be combined in a mixing dish.
- Combine well after mixing.
- Roll little amounts of the mixture into balls.
- Before serving, store the energy balls in the refrigerator for at least 30 minutes in an airtight container.

Guacamole:

Ingredients:

- 2 ripe avocados
- 1 small tomato, diced
- 1/4 cup red onion, finely chopped
- 1 jalapeno pepper, seeded and minced (optional)
- Juice of 1 lime
- Handful of fresh cilantro, chopped
- Salt and pepper to taste

steps

- Remove the pit from the avocados, then scoop out the meat into a basin.
- With a fork, mash the avocados until the required consistency is achieved.
- Add the minced tomato, red onion, cilantro, lime juice, and salt and pepper to taste.
- To thoroughly incorporate all ingredients, stir well.
- If necessary, taste and adjust the seasoning.
- Serve with veggie sticks or whole-wheat tortilla chips.

Roasted Chickpeas:

Ingredients:

- 1 can chickpeas, drained and rinsed
- 1 tablespoon olive oil
- 1 teaspoon paprika
- 1/2 teaspoon cumin
- 1/2 teaspoon garlic powder
- Salt to taste

steps

- Set the oven's temperature to 400°F (200°C).
- Using a paper towel, pat dry the chickpeas to get rid of extra moisture.
- Chickpeas should be well coated in a bowl with olive oil, paprika, cumin, garlic powder, and salt.
- On a baking sheet, distribute the chickpeas in a single layer.
- Bake the chickpeas for 25 to 30 minutes, or until they are crisp and golden brown.
- Before serving as a crispy snack, let them cool.

Veggie Sushi Rolls:

Ingredients:
- Nori sheets (seaweed)

- Cooked sushi rice
- Assorted vegetables (such as cucumber, avocado, carrots, bell peppers)
- Soy sauce or tamari (for dipping)

Steps

- On a bamboo sushi mat or a fresh kitchen towel, spread a sheet of nori.
- Over the nori, spread cooked sushi rice evenly, leaving a thin border at the top.
- Vegetables should be arranged in thin strips along the center of the rice.
- Apply little pressure to firmly roll the nori using a sushi mat or cloth, holding everything together.
- To seal the roll, lightly wet the top border of the nori.
- Use a sharp knife to cut the sushi roll into bite-sized pieces.
- Serve with tamari or soy sauce for dipping.

Baked Sweet Potato Fries:

Ingredients:

- Sweet potatoes, peeled and cut into fries
- Olive oil
- Salt and pepper to taste
- Optional: paprika, garlic powder, or other seasonings of choice

steps

- A baking sheet should be lined with parchment paper and the oven should be preheated to 425°F (220°C).
- Sweet potato fries should be mixed with olive oil, salt, pepper, and any additional ingredients in a bowl.
- On the baking sheet that has been prepared, spread the fries in a single layer.
- Fries should be baked for 20 to 25 minutes, turning them over halfway through, until crispy and browned.
- Before serving, take them out of the oven and allow them to cool somewhat.

Caprese Skewers:

Ingredients:

- Cherry tomatoes
- Fresh mozzarella balls
- Fresh basil leaves
- Balsamic glaze or reduction
- Skewers or toothpicks

steps

- On a skewer or toothpick, arrange a mozzarella ball, a cherry tomato, and some fresh basil.
- Continue until all the ingredients have been utilized.
- On a serving dish, arrange the skewers.
- Apply a glaze or reduction of balsamic.
- Use as a light and energizing starter.

Cucumber and Hummus Bites:

Ingredients:

- English cucumber
- Hummus
- Cherry tomatoes, halved
- Fresh dill or parsley for garnish

steps

- Make thick circles out of the cucumber.
- Create a little depression in each cucumber round using a small spoon or melon baller.
- Put a dab of hummus in the depression.
- Add a cherry tomato cut in half on top.
- Add fresh parsley or dill as a garnish.
- Serve the bite-sized cucumber and hummus appetizers from a plate.

These dishes cater to a variety of tastes and preferences by offering a variety of flavors and textures. Try out these healthy snack and appetizer suggestions, and feel free to make them your own. Enjoy!

Chapter 7

Satisfying Sides and Accompaniments

The value of sides and accompaniments in constructing a balanced and fulfilling dinner cannot be emphasized. In addition to enhancing the tastes and textures of the main course, these supplemental dishes offer a chance to include a range of nutrient-dense products. Focusing on sides and accompaniments that are rich with nutrients that combat inflammation is essential for ensuring good health and well-being in the context of an anti-inflammatory diet for seniors.

Colorful Roasted and Grilled Vegetables: Vegetables may be roasted or grilled to bring out their natural tastes while retaining their nutritious worth. Anti-inflammatory herbs and spices like turmeric, ginger, and garlic can be used to season colorful vegetables like bell peppers, zucchini, eggplant, and carrots. They make a delightful and colorful side dish when drizzled with a little olive oil and roasted till soft. They go well with a variety of main entrees.

Wholesome whole grains and salads made with ancient grains: Including whole grains in sides and salads gives a meal a filling and healthy component. In addition to being high in fiber, choices like quinoa, brown rice, farro, and bulgur also offer necessary vitamins and minerals. Grain salads with various veggies, herbs, and a tangy vinaigrette may produce a light and satisfying side dish. These salads are adaptable and practical for senior lunches because they may be eaten cold or at room temperature.

Delicious sides and casseroles made with legumes: Legumes, such as beans, lentils, and chickpeas, are nutritious powerhouses that have a host of health advantages. They are great providers of fiber, a variety of vitamins, and minerals, as well as plant-based protein. Legume-based sides and casseroles may be a filling and satisfying complement to any dinner. In addition to promoting fullness, dishes like bean salads, lentil soups, and chickpea stews also assist digestive health and blood sugar regulation.

Anti-inflammatory Sauces, Dressings, and Condiments: Enhancing your meals with tasty and healthy sauces, dressings, and condiments may improve the eating experience and offer extra health advantages. By choosing homemade alternatives, you can manage the components and stay away from processed chemicals. For instance, a creamy avocado dressing may be drizzled over salads or served as a dip and is created with avocado, lemon juice, herbs, and a little olive oil. Similar to how homemade tomato sauce may enhance the flavor of pasta meals or roasted vegetables, anti-inflammatory herbs like basil and oregano can do the same.

A senior's anti-inflammatory diet should include gratifying sides and accompaniments since doing so improves the meal as a whole and guarantees that it is well-balanced and nutrient-dense. Seniors may strengthen their immune systems, lessen chronic inflammation, and enhance their general health by focusing on components with anti-inflammatory qualities.

The special dietary requirements and preferences of older citizens should be taken into account while making sides and accompaniments. To satisfy any dietary restrictions or sensitivities, it could be required to modify the spices, textures, and cooking techniques. Working with a healthcare professional or certified dietitian can also offer individualized advice on serving sizes and certain nutritional issues.

Seniors may have a varied and healthy eating experience that supports their general health and well-being by adopting a choice of pleasing sides and accompaniments that are both delicious and anti-inflammatory.

Chapter 8

Sweet Treats and Desserts

One of life's basic joys is indulging in desserts and other sweet delicacies. There is something innately delicious about finishing a meal with something sweet, whether it be decadent chocolates or fruity treats. Traditional sweets, however, frequently include components that might exacerbate inflammation and other health issues. Fortunately, by adopting a thoughtful attitude and using anti-inflammatory components, you may indulge in delectable sweets that not only sate your desires but also promote your general wellbeing.

The emphasis is on employing products that have proven anti-inflammatory effects when making sweet delights with an anti-inflammatory twist. Fruits, nuts, seeds, whole grains, and spices are some of these nutrients. These foods are brimming with healthy substances including phytochemicals and antioxidants. You may increase your desserts' nutritious content and eat guilt-free by adding these ingredients.

Fruit-based sweets are a common type of anti-inflammatory dessert. In addition to offering a natural sweetness, fresh fruits like berries, mangoes, and citrus fruits are also a great source of fiber, vitamins, and minerals. They may be added to a variety of sweets, including fruit compotes, fruit parfaits, and fruit salads. Baked fruits with a drizzle of honey, a sprinkling of cinnamon, and other delectable ingredients make a warm and welcoming dessert.

Another key ingredient in making satiating and anti-inflammatory sweets is nuts and seeds. They are great providers of fiber, protein, and good fats. These nutrients, which range from chia seeds and flaxseeds to almonds and walnuts, can be utilized in a number of different ways. For instance, you might use a combination of nuts, seeds, dried fruit, and natural sweeteners like dates or maple syrup to make your own energy balls or granola bars. These delights deliver a pleasant crunch in addition to a flavorful explosion.

When making healthy treats, whole grains are essential. Instead of using refined white flour, choose whole grain flours like whole wheat or spelt flour to get more fiber and other nutrients. A healthier alternative of traditional treats like whole grain cookies, muffins, or cakes may be made with this. You may experiment with other flours to give your sweets a distinctive touch while keeping them gluten-free, such as almond or coconut flour.

Another approach to boost the nutritional content of your sweet sweets is by adding anti-inflammatory spices. In addition to adding delicious tastes, spices like cinnamon, turmeric, ginger, and cloves also have anti-inflammatory and antioxidant qualities. Various dessert dishes, such as spiced fruit compotes, turmeric golden milk puddings, or ginger-flavored biscuits, can use these spices. Your pastries will taste even better thanks to the fragrant warmth of these spices, which also give them depth and complexity.

It is recommended to use natural sweeteners rather than processed sugars to sweeten your sweets. Natural sweeteners that give sweetness and some nutritional advantages include honey, maple syrup, and coconut sugar. They are less processed and have small levels of antioxidants and minerals. However, it's crucial to use these sweeteners sparingly because overusing them can still have an adverse effect on blood sugar levels.

A variety of delicious desserts may be created by experimenting with different combinations of these anti-inflammatory components. There are various options for making desserts that not only sate your sweet taste but also promote your general health, from hydrating smoothies and puddings to nourishing baked products and frozen delicacies.

In conclusion, indulging in sweet snacks and desserts need not be a sin. Fruits, nuts, seeds, whole grains, and spices are anti-inflammatory foods that may be used to make delectable sweets that enhance wellbeing. These sweets offer a harmony of tastes, textures, and nutrition, letting you splurge guilt-free. Discover the thrill of feeding your health while satisfying your sweet tooth by exploring the world of anti-inflammatory sweets.